Herbal TEA RECIPES

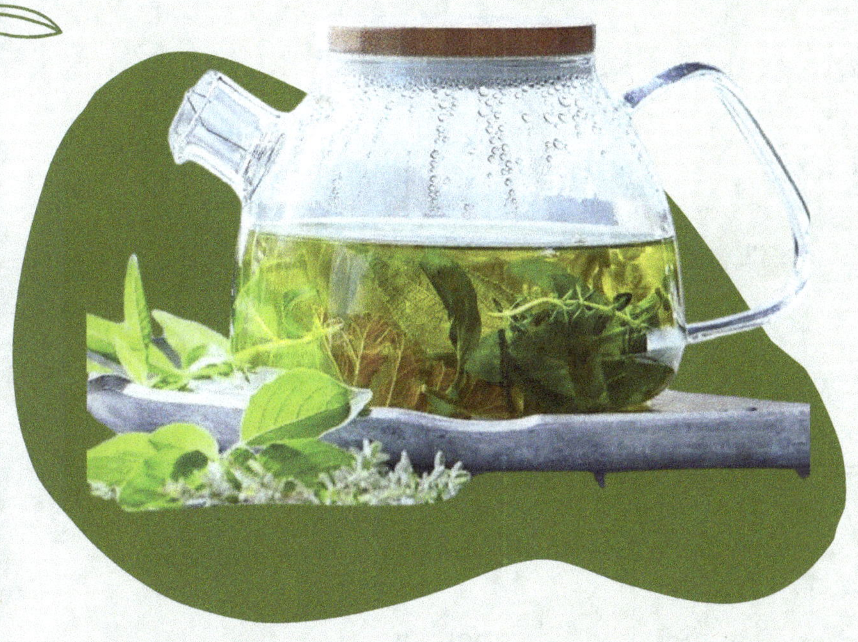

Boost Immunity, Reduce Stress, and Improve Sleep

TABLE CONTENT

Rooibos & pear tea   32

Cinnamon tea   35

Lemon & ginger tea   38

Lavender Tea   41

Jasmine & ginger tea   44

Mint & mango iced green tea   47

Matcha with vanilla   50

Blueberry & mint iced tea   53

Chai tea   56

Sage Tea   59

Iced hibiscus tea   62

Turmeric tea   65

Rosemary & orange iced tea   68

Thank you

Introduction

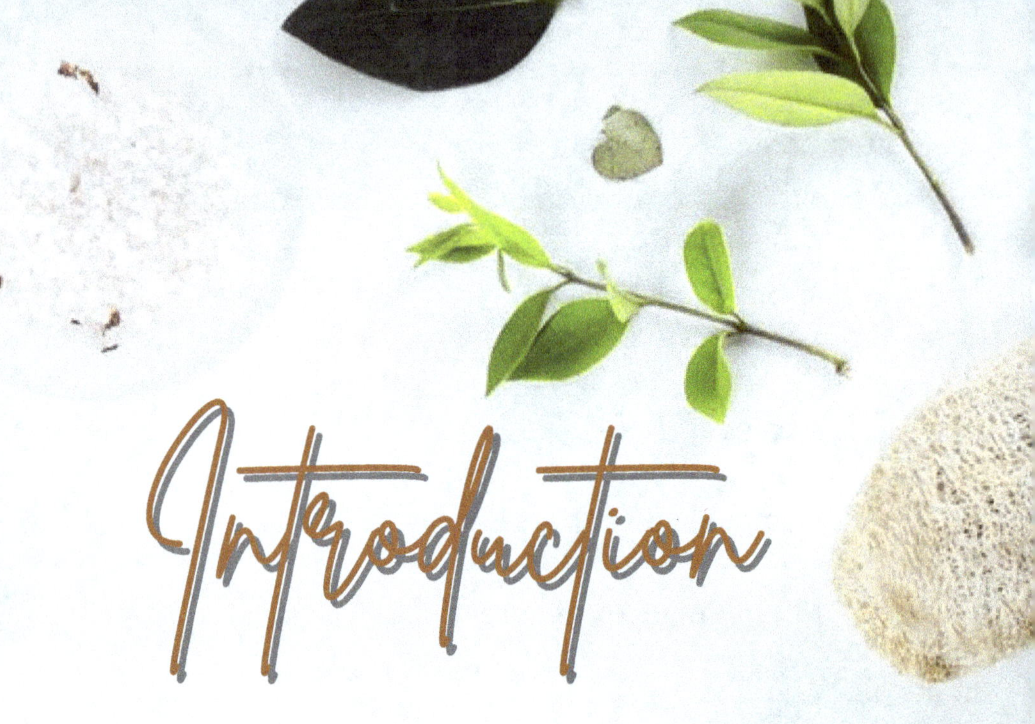

In our fast-paced world, feeling overwhelmed, depleted, and sleep-deprived is all too common. We crave natural solutions to bolster our well-being and rediscover a sense of calm. Enter the world of herbal teas – a simple yet powerful tool for nurturing both body and mind.

This book, "Herbal Tea Recipes: Boost Immunity, Reduce Stress, and Improve Sleep," is your guide to harnessing the power of nature's bounty. Within these pages, you'll discover a collection of delicious and effective tea blends designed to support your specific needs.

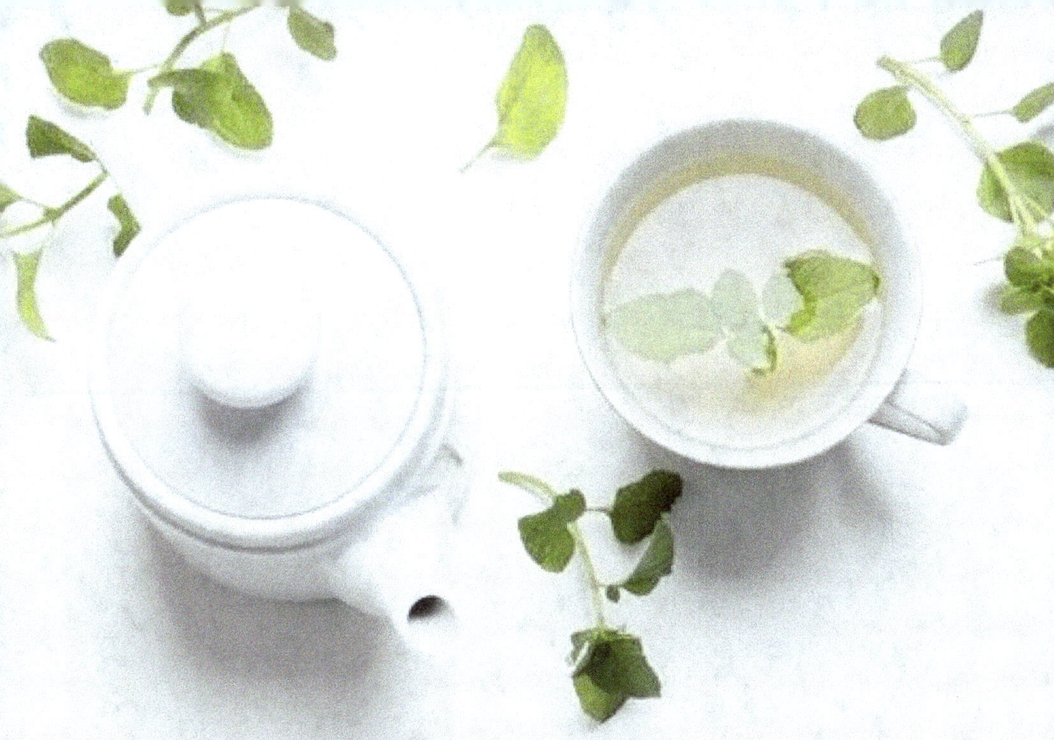

Whether you're seeking to fortify your immune system, quiet a restless mind, or drift off to a deeper sleep, there's a perfect cup of herbal magic waiting to be brewed. We'll delve into the science behind each ingredient, explaining how different herbs work to promote optimal health.

But this book goes beyond just recipes. It's an invitation to cultivate a mindful tea ritual. Learn tips for selecting high-quality ingredients, brewing methods for optimal flavor, and creating a relaxing atmosphere to enjoy your cup.
So, put the kettle on, gather your favorite mug, and embark on a journey of self-care with the gentle guidance of herbal teas. Let each sip be a step towards a stronger, calmer, and more restful you.

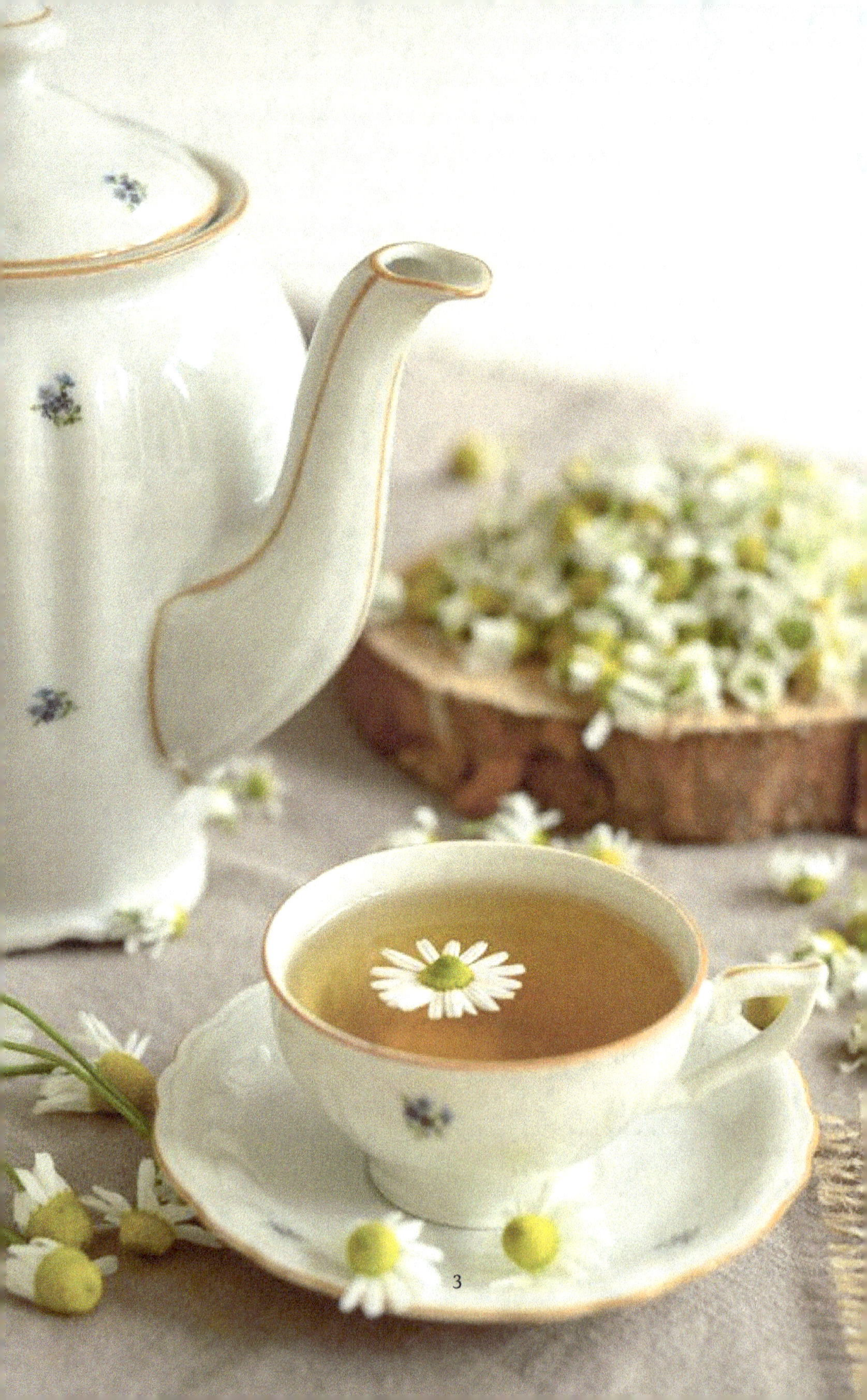

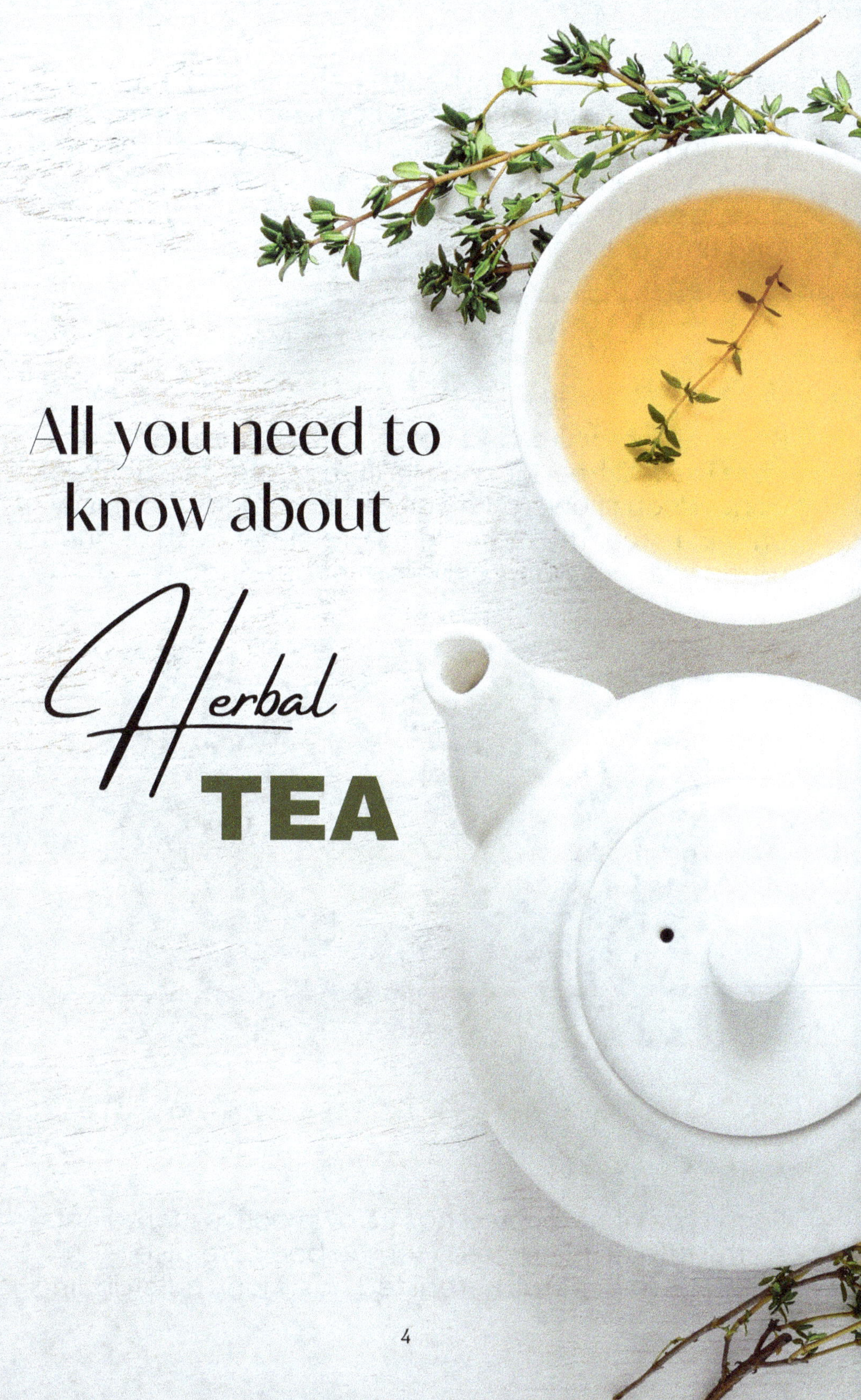

All you need to know about

Herbal TEA

Herbal tea offers many health benefits such as preventing cancer, diabetes, cardiovascular disease, reducing anxiety, insomnia,... However, you should also be careful when choosing herbal teas. , time and dose, as some can cause side effects if used for a long time or taken in excessive amounts.

1. What is herbal tea? What is the difference from green tea?

Black, green, white, and oolong teas are all derived from the tea tree. Meanwhile, herbal teas are derived from various flowers, leaves or spices and are mostly caffeine-free. The ingredients are either fresh or dried, mixed with hot water or boiled for drinking.

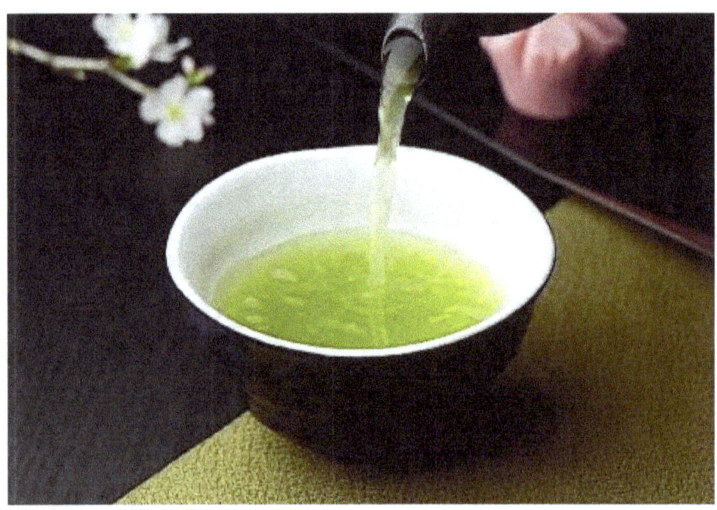

2. What are the benefits of drinking herbal tea?

Each type of herbal tea has its own active ingredients, so the effects of each tea for the body are also different. In general, herbal tea has many outstanding health

benefits including:
Against liver, cervical, colon, lymphatic or lung cancer,...; Reduce the risk of diabetes and its complications; Prevent the risk of neurodegenerative diseases such as Alzheimer's; Increases fat metabolism, reduces fat, has the ability to support weight loss; Protect liver, clear heat, detoxify; Improve the immune system; Reduce fever, relieve cough and sore throat; Sedative, stress relief.

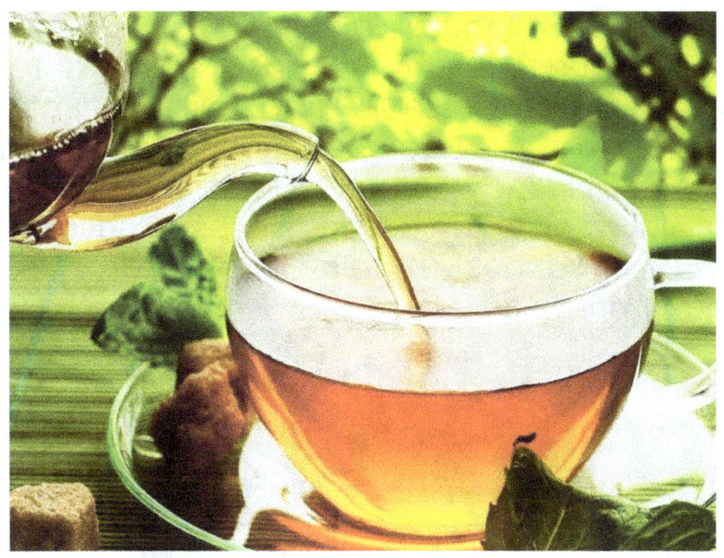

3. Is drinking herbal tea good?

Rooibos tea:

Rooibos tea, also known as red tea, is native to South Africa. The ingredient does not contain caffeine and is believed to have antioxidant effects. Based on scientific studies, this tea has immune-boosting and cancer-preventing effects. Cardiovascular and diabetes benefits are under review. You should consult your doctor before using rooibos tea if you have hormone-sensitive cancer or are undergoing chemotherapy. Chamomile Tea: Has been used for centuries to soothe upset stomachs, bloating, diarrhea, insomnia, and anxiety. However, there are currently new studies demonstrating its anxiety-reducing effects, for other benefits that have not been specifically studied. Chamomile tea is contraindicated in people who are allergic to ragweed plants and are taking blood-thinning medications such as warfarin. Rosehip Tea: Rosehip tea is extracted from the bark of the rosehip seed, which is a great source of vitamin C with anti-inflammatory and antioxidant properties. Some even claim it helps ease the pain of arthritis, but more research is needed. Rosehip tea is relatively safe, with only a few cases of allergic reactions or stomach upset when drinking the tea. Peppermint tea: Peppermint tea is often used in cases of upset stomach, headaches, irritable bowel syndrome and respiratory problems.

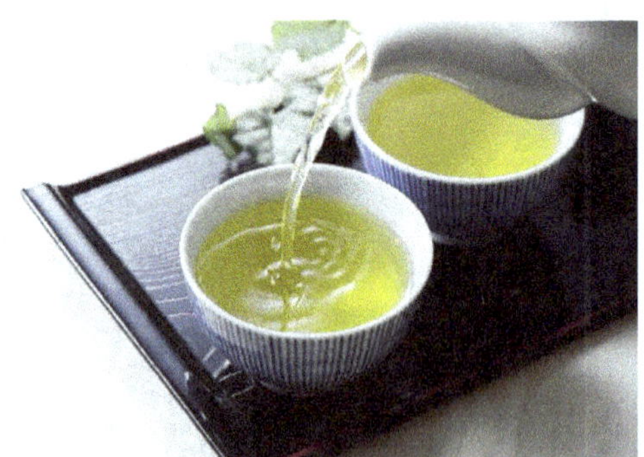

Although it has been used medicinally for centuries, there is little research supporting its health benefits. This tea is safe, so you can try or simply enjoy the cool taste of mint. Ginger tea:
Mainly used in the treatment of stomach upset and nausea. In addition, you can also use it to increase appetite, relieve pain from arthritis or prevent colds. Some studies have found evidence of an anti-nausea

effect, but other benefits are still to be explored. Ginger tea is considered safe, but if you are pregnant, you should consult your doctor before using it as a regular drink. Lemon Balm tea (Lemon Balm): According to folk tradition, perilla tea has the effect of reducing anxiety, insomnia and there is some evidence to prove this. As for the memory-improving effect, more research is needed. This tea can cause nausea and stomach upset, so be careful when drinking too much or
for a long time. Milk thistle and dandelion tea:
Milk thistle and dandelion tea are used for people with liver and bile diseases. Dandelion tea is not usually harmful to health, except for people who are allergic to plants with yellow flowers. Milk thistle tea has the main ingredient silymarin, which studies have shown to be effective in reducing the symptoms of hepatitis C.

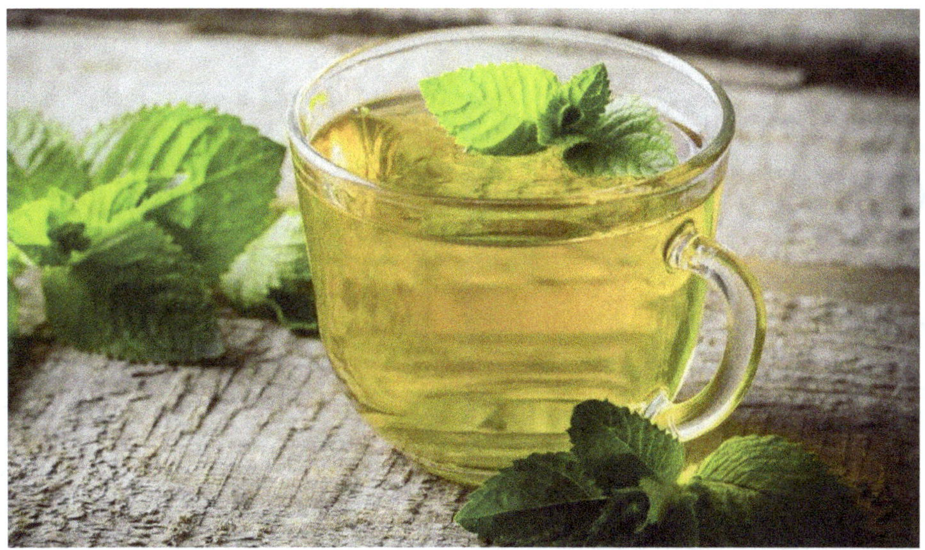

Hibiscus Tea:
Hibiscus flower tea originated in ancient Egypt, from a red flower rich in antioxidants. Some studies have found it to lower blood pressure and cholesterol. This is a safe tea, you can drink it in moderation without harming your

health. Echinacea tea:
Echinacea also known as coneflower, is a remedy used to treat colds thanks to its immune-boosting effects. However, there are currently not many studies proving its benefits. If you are pregnant, have allergies or asthma, or are on medication, you should not use this tea. Sage tea:
Used for centuries in the treatment of stomach problems, sore throats, depression and memory loss. However, research on the health benefits of this herb is still limited. Most types of sage tea are safe to consume, with the exception of a few that contain thujone, which can affect the nervous system. Passionflower tea:
Has the effect of alleviating anxiety and helping to treat insomnia. However, you should not drink this tea if you

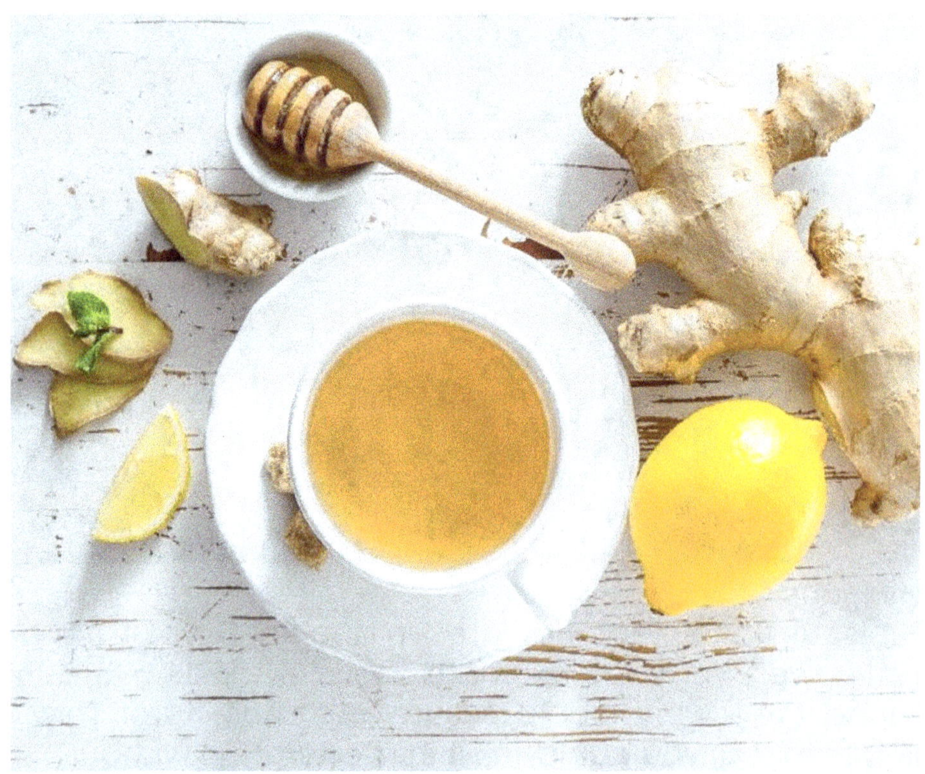

are pregnant as it can cause side effects such as drowsiness, dizziness and confusion. Passion fruit tea may also affect the action of certain medications, such

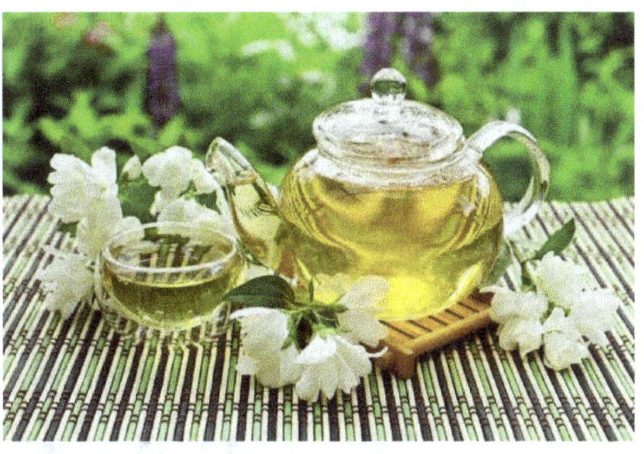

as pentobarbital and benzodiazepines. Turmeric tea: Used by some people to treat kidney stones and bloating, but there are currently no studies to support this. Animal studies have shown it to prevent cancer and reduce inflammation, but human studies are still needed to accurately assess its effects. If you are undergoing chemotherapy, you should not drink turmeric tea because it can interfere with the treatment process. Valerian tea:
Women use valerian tea to relieve symptoms of menopause, in addition, it is also used in the treatment of insomnia, anxiety or depression. Some studies have demonstrated the sedative effects of tea, however, should not be used for a long time or in combination with alcohol or sedatives, to avoid harm to health. Kava tea:
Kava is a plant in the pepper family, native to the South Pacific, commonly known as a tonic with proven anxiety-reducing effects. However, researchers have also discovered liver side effects such as yellowing or dry, scaly skin with long-term use. The FDA has issued a warning about the risks associated with using this tea and some countries are trying to remove it from the market.

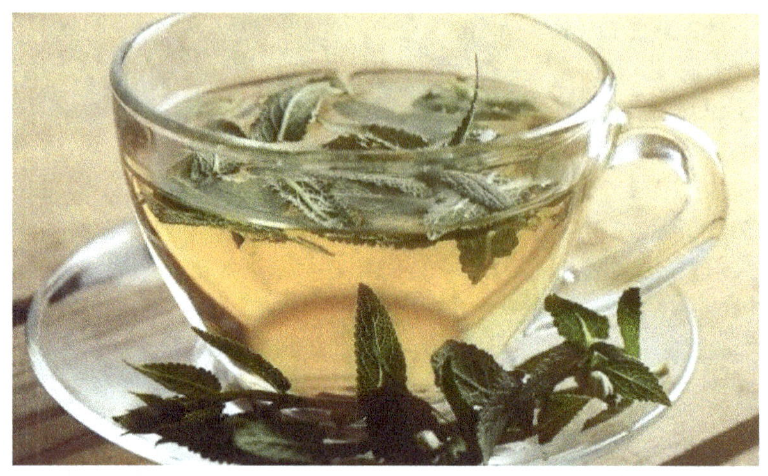

Overall, herbal tea has many outstanding health benefits. However, you should consult your doctor about herbal teas, timing and dosage, as some can cause side effects if used for a long time or taken in excessive amounts.

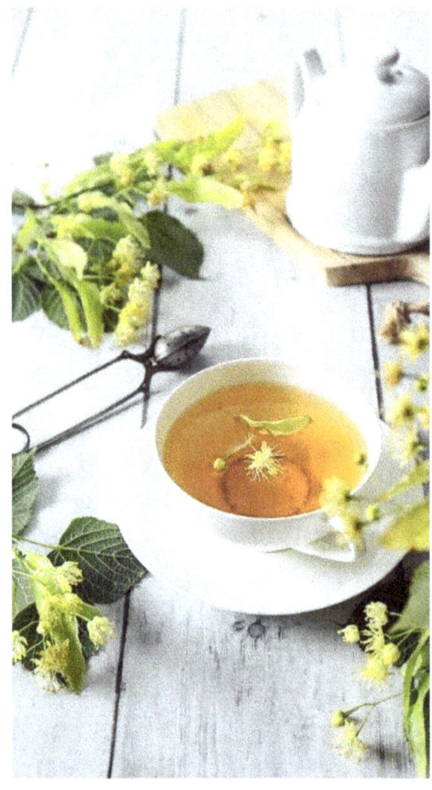

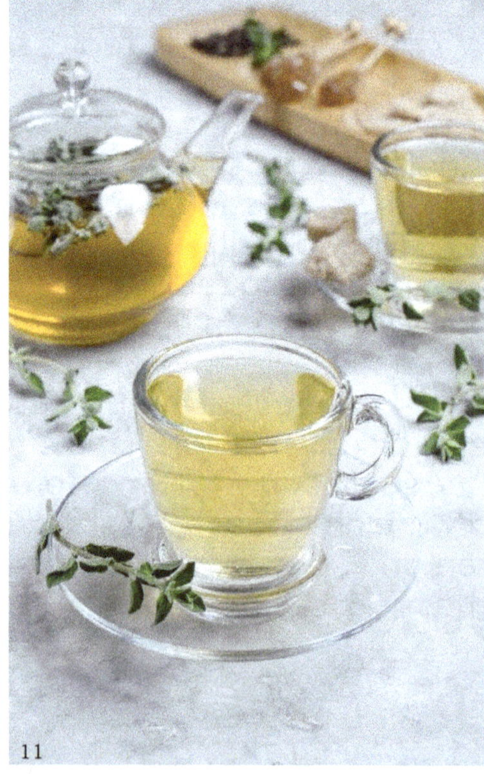

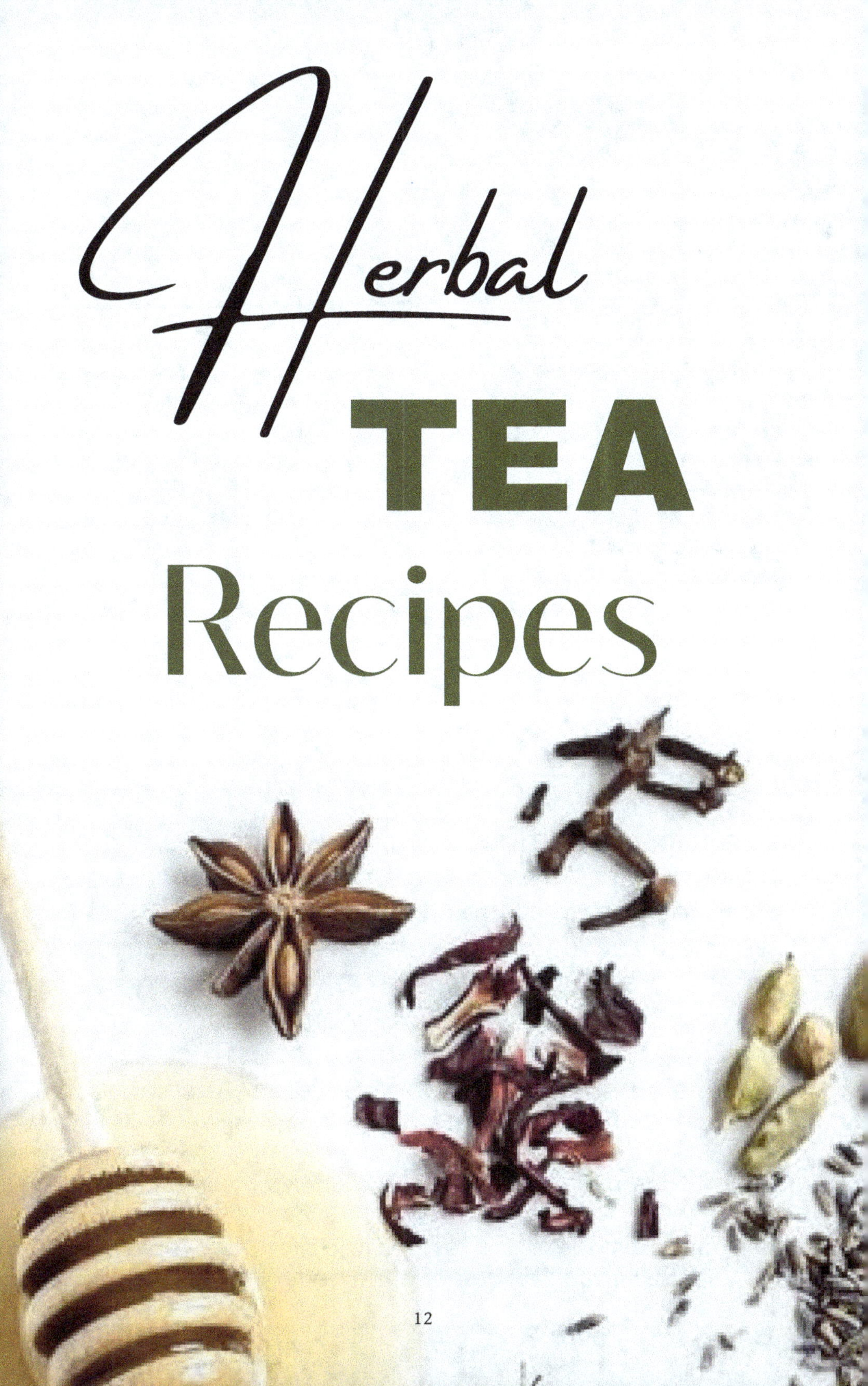

Herbal **TEA** Recipes

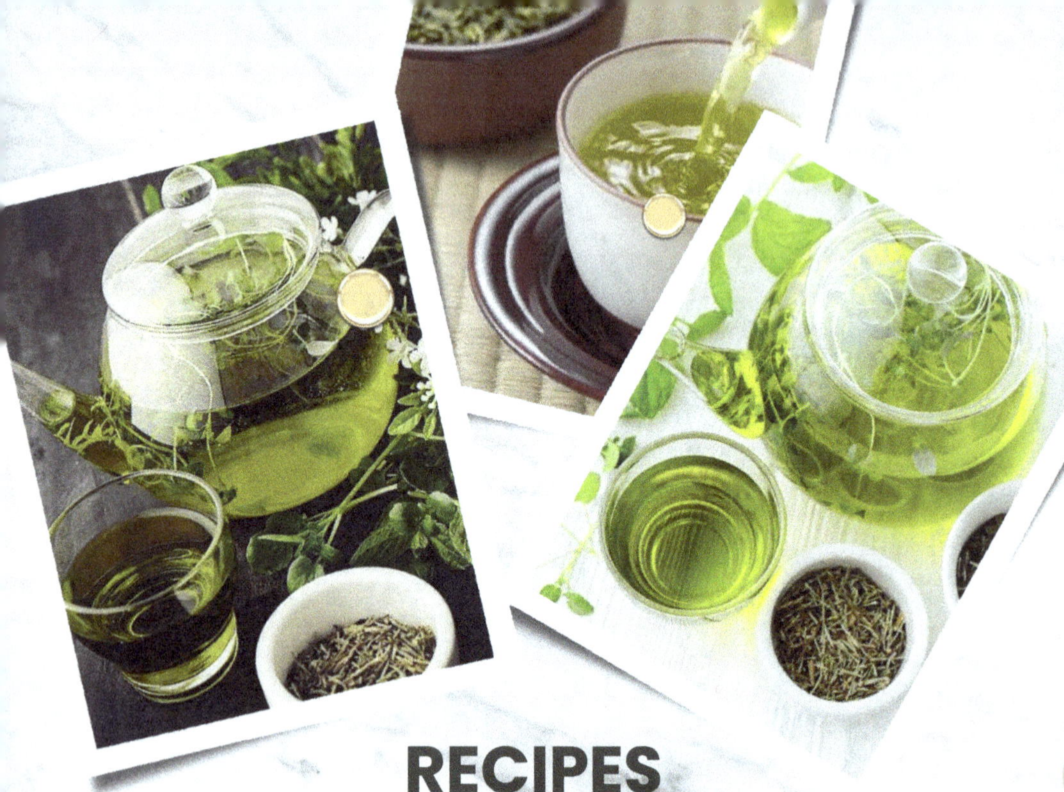

RECODES

Herbal Tea

Settle in for an aromatic pot of fiery ginger tea, or start of the day with a fresh, minty brew. Our favourite easy tea recipes are perfect for accompanying your favourite treats or giving you a boost in the afternoon. Whether you want to elevate a simple cup of green tea or create a refreshing, fruity blend that's all your own, take some inspiration from our best recipes. We have everything from warming pots to refreshing iced options for when the sun is shining.

Make a batch of easy biscuits to munch with your cuppa, too.
Check out more of our tea recipes and afternoon tea recipes for inspiration on creating the perfect tea party.

THYME TEA

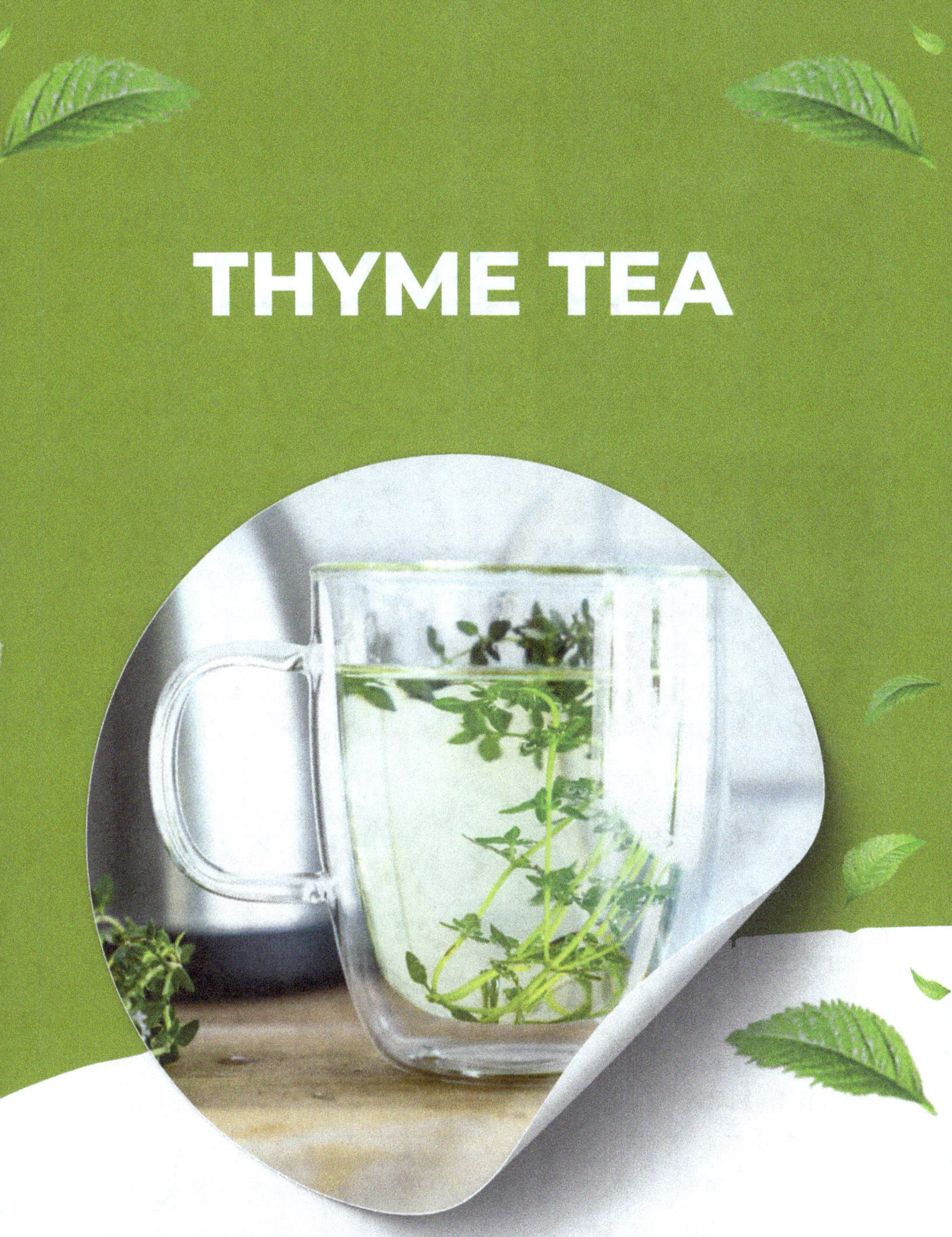

Thyme tea is a restorative herbal tea made with just boiling water and fresh thyme! Just 5 minutes to the perfect cup of tea.

Thyme Tea

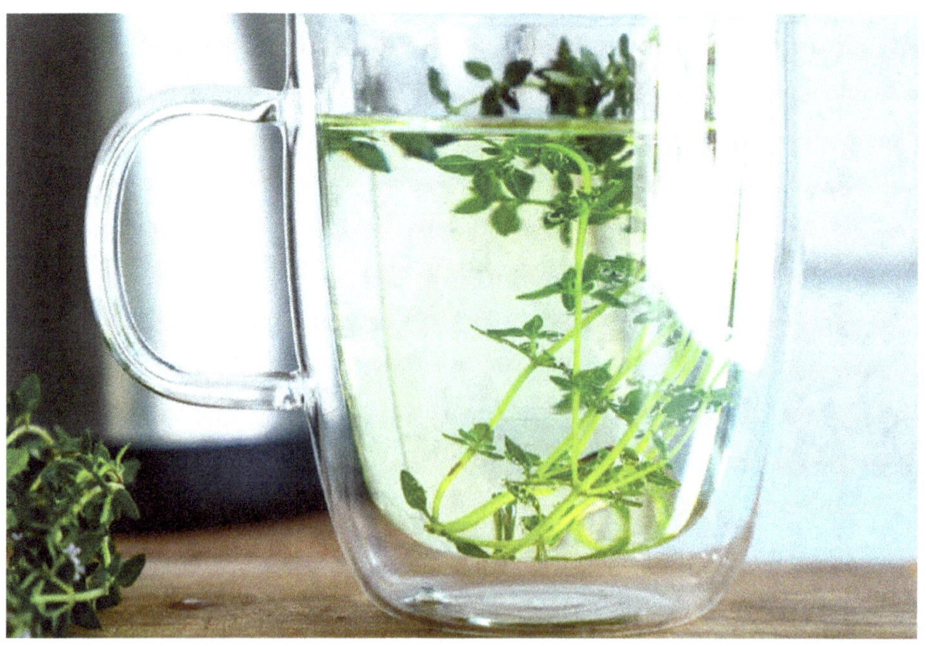

Prep Time : 5 mins

Level : Easy

Servings : 1 drink

Ingredients :

- 8 to 10 fresh thyme sprigs (standard or lemon thyme)
- Boiling water

Method :

1 Bring the water to a boil.

2 Wash the thyme thoroughly.

Thyme Tea

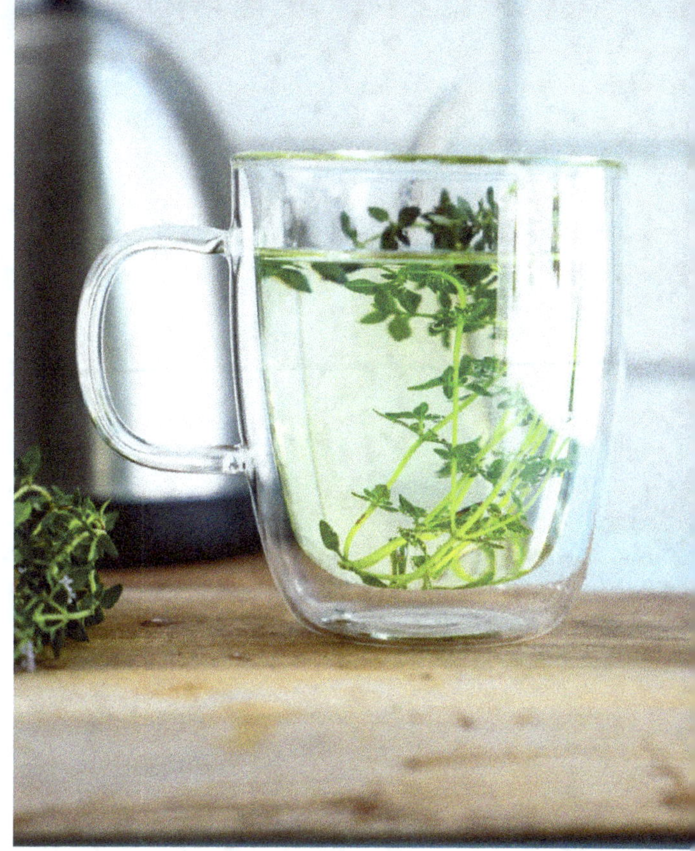

Method :

3 Place the thyme sprigs in a mug, and pour over the boiling water. Allow the thyme to steep for 5 minutes. Remove the thyme and enjoy. (Alternate method: If you prefer, you can also chop the thyme leaves and place them in a tea strainer before steeping.)

Thyme tea is restorative, delicious, and takes just 5 minutes to steep into a flavorful tea. When we tried this herbal tea for the first time, we were astounded by the flavor. Thyme tea tastes herby, fragrant and satisfying. It's a fun way to make DIY tea, and makes drinking water much more exciting.

SMOKY GINGER & HONEY TEA

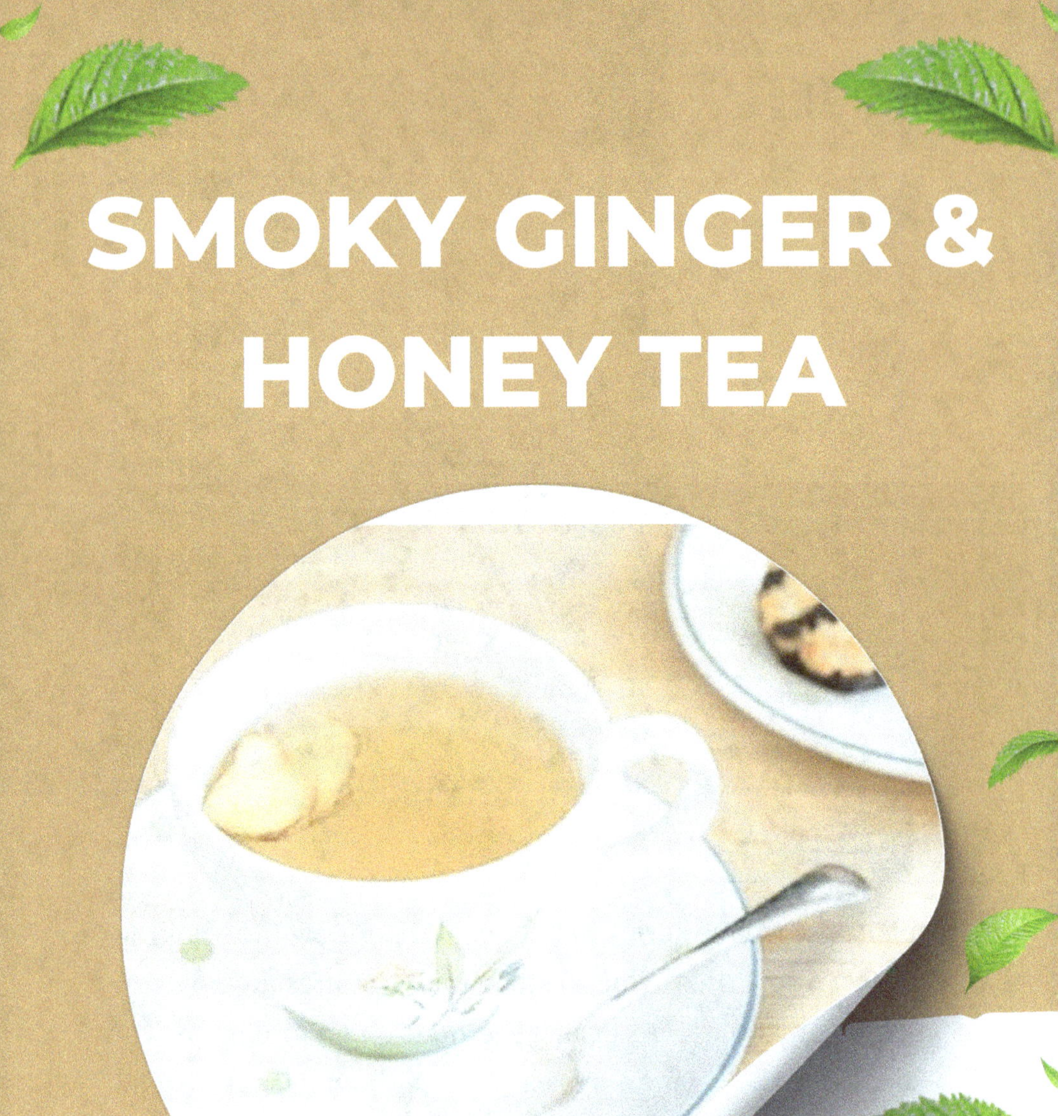

Swap your regular cup of tea for this smoky blend, which combines the flavour of lapsang souchong loose tea leaves with root ginger, green tea and honey

Smoky ginger & honey tea

Prep Time : 5 mins

Level : Easy

Servings : Serves 1

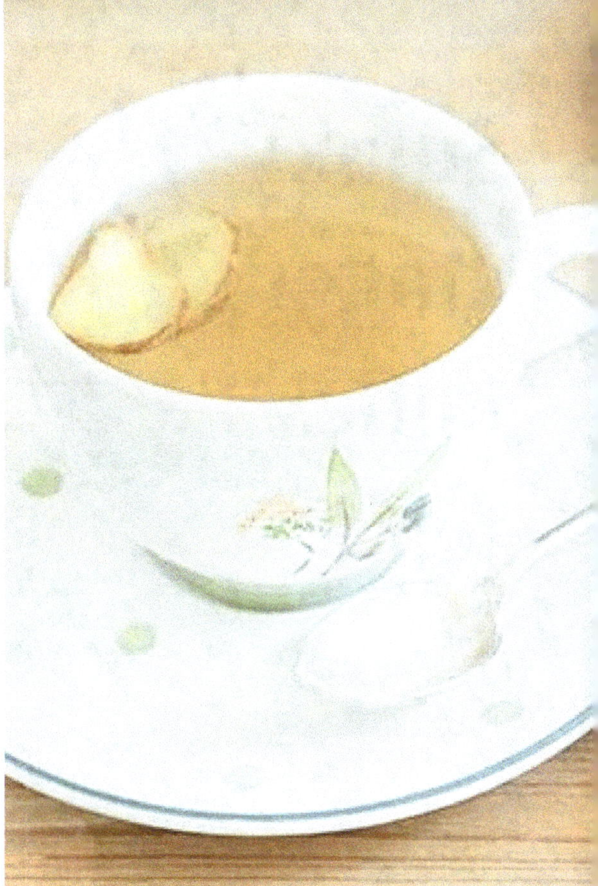

Ingredients :

- thumbsized piece of root ginger, sliced
- ½ tsp lapsang souchong tea leaves
- ½ tsp green tea leaves
- ½-1 tsp honey

Method :

1. Set a slice of ginger aside and put the rest into your teapot, then add both types of tea leaves. Fill your cup with boiling water then pour it into the teapot – this allows the water to cool down a little bit first.

Smoky ginger & honey tea

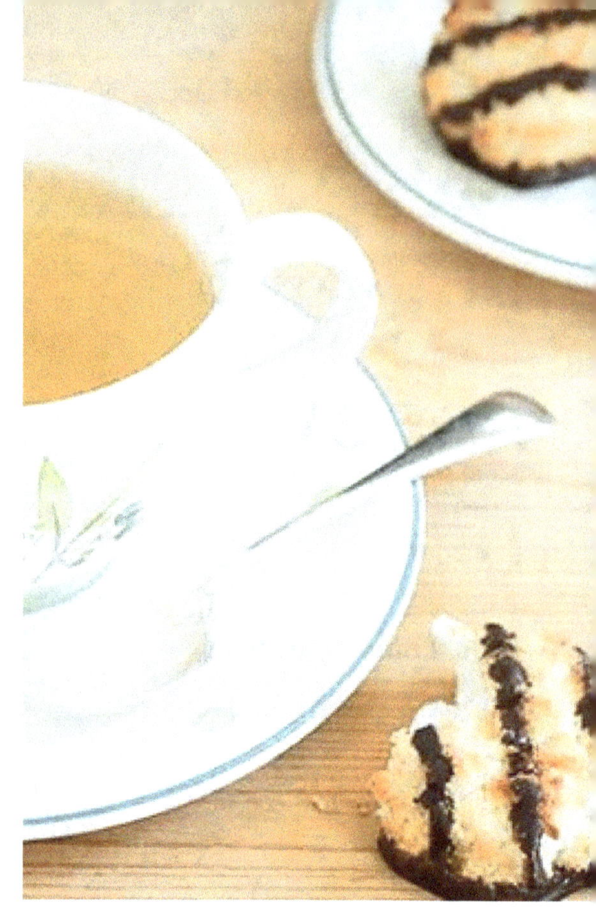

Method :

2   Leave the tea to brew for 1 min then strain into your cup. Add honey to taste and the reserved ginger slice.

FRESH MINT TEA

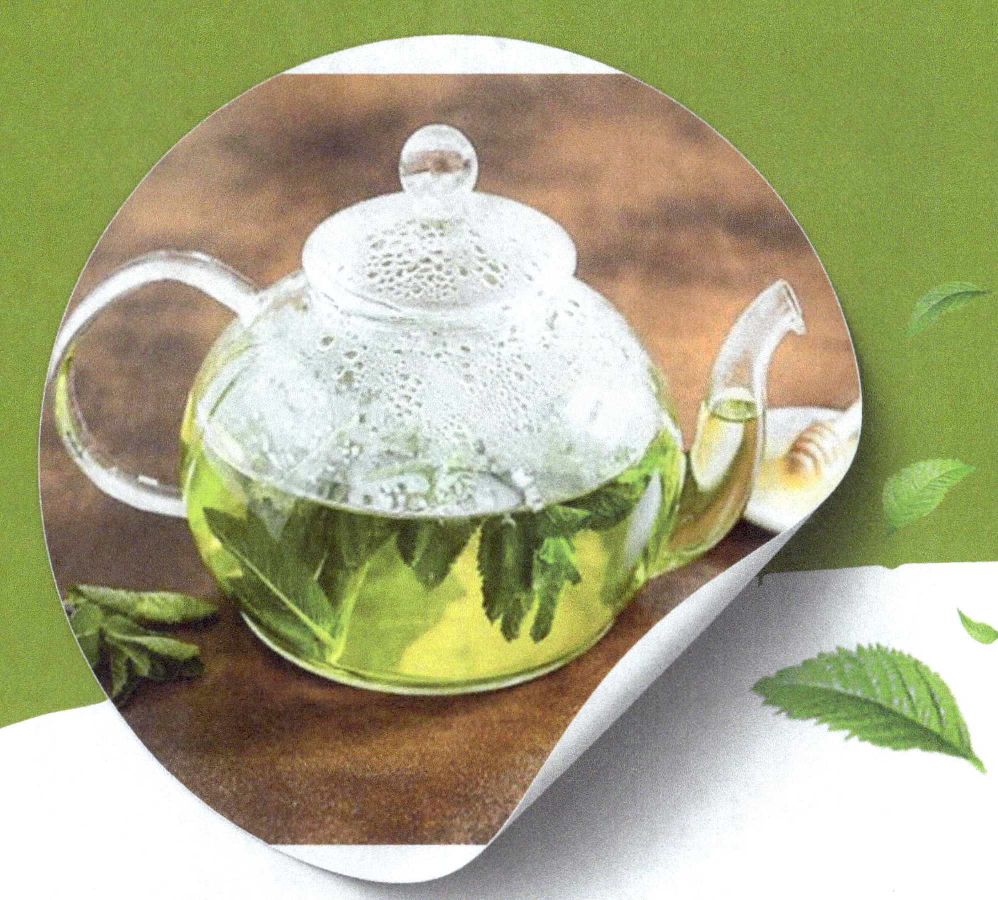

Grab a handful of fresh mint leaves and pour over boiling water to release its wonderful flavour and scent. Sweeten the tea with honey according to taste

Fresh mint tea

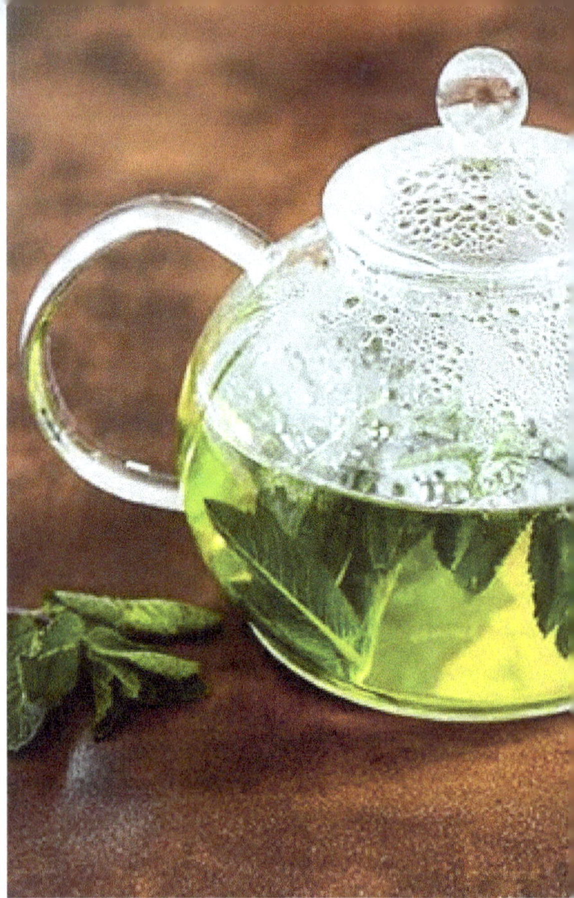

Prep Time : 5 mins

Level : Easy

Servings : Makes one 500-600ml pot (serves 1-2)

Ingredients :

- handful of fresh mint (around ½ a pack)
- honey to taste

Our Most Popular Alternative

- Harissa aubergine wedges with tahini & mint yogurt

Method :

1. Take a few leaves of the mint in one hand and sharply clap your other hand on top, then drop the leaves into a teapot or cafetiere. Repeat with the rest of the mint, saving a few small sprigs for each glass as a garnish.

Fresh mint tea

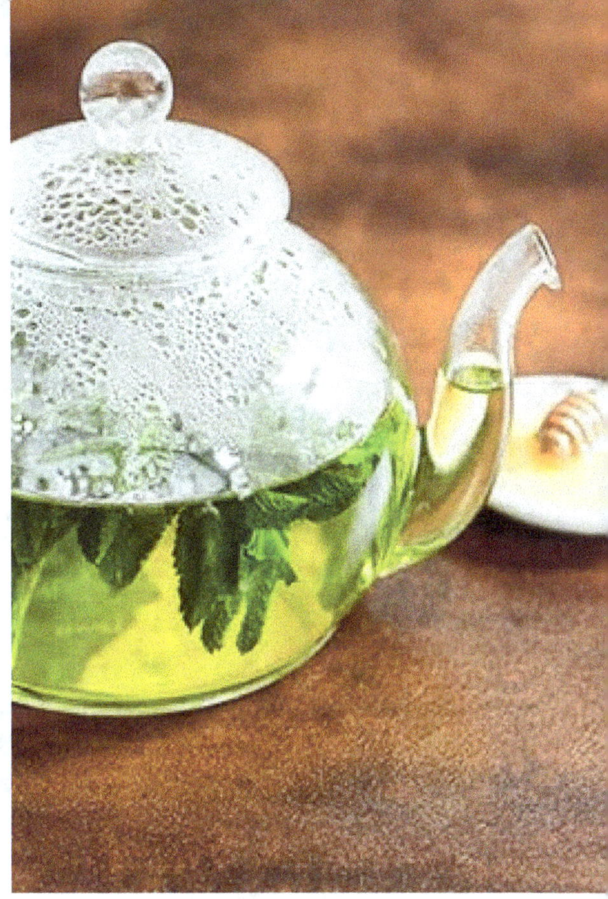

Method :

2 Fill up the pot with boiling water and let it infuse for 2-3 mins or until the liquid starts to take on a slight pale yellow/green hue. Strain the tea into cups or heatproof glasses and sweeten with honey to taste. Drop the reserved mint into the cups to decorate if you like.

Refresh your tastebuds with a pot of vibrant green fresh mint tea. Just grab a handful of mint leaves and add boiling water to release its distinctive flavour and scent. Sweeten it according to your own taste with honey. You'll never go back to teabags once you've tried the real thing.

CAMOMILE TEA WITH HONEY

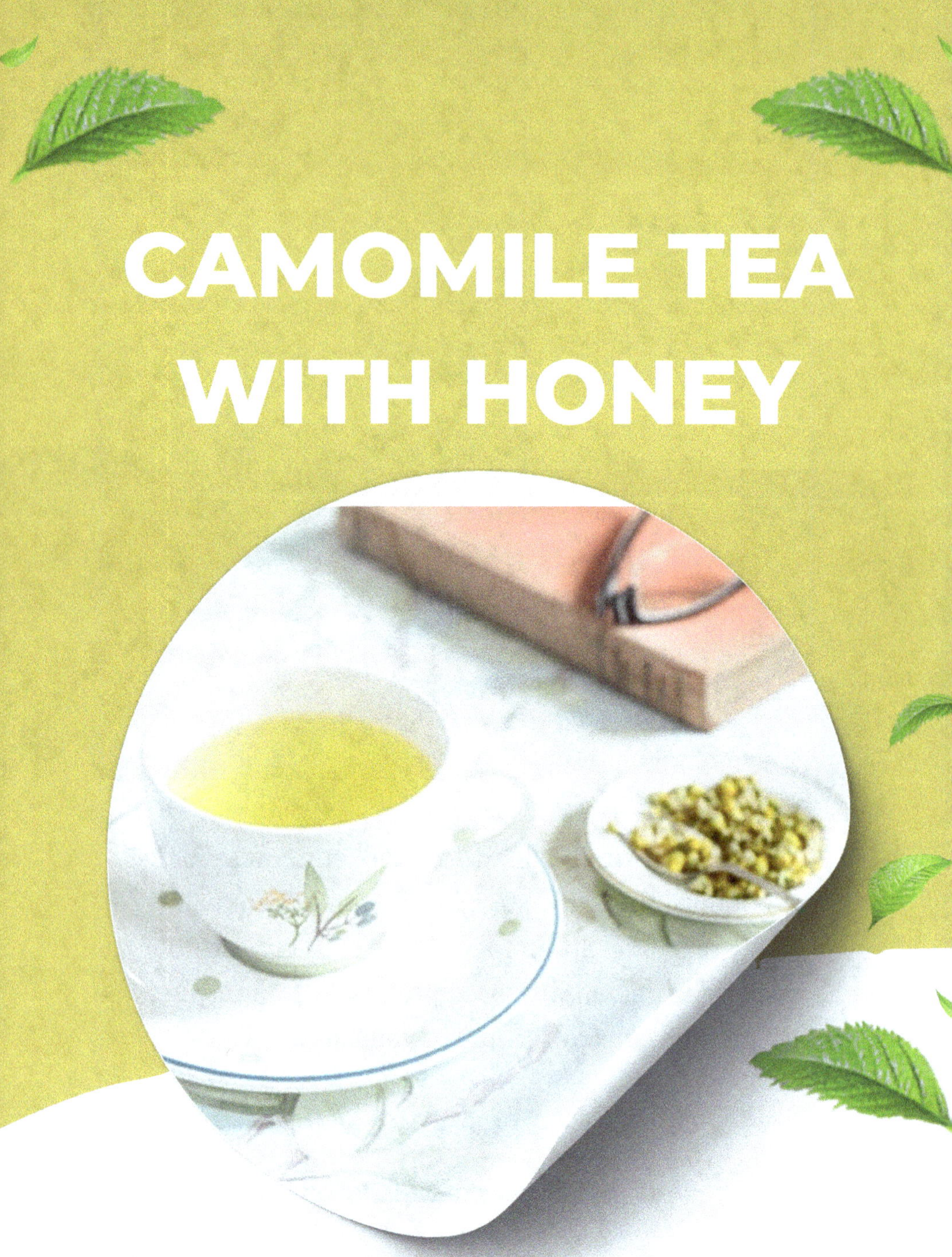

Combine dried camomile flowers with aromatic lavender and honey to make this wonderfully calming tea, perfect in the morning or for winding down in the evening

Camomile tea with honey

Prep Time : 5 mins

Level : Easy

Servings : Makes one 500-600ml pot (serves 1-2)

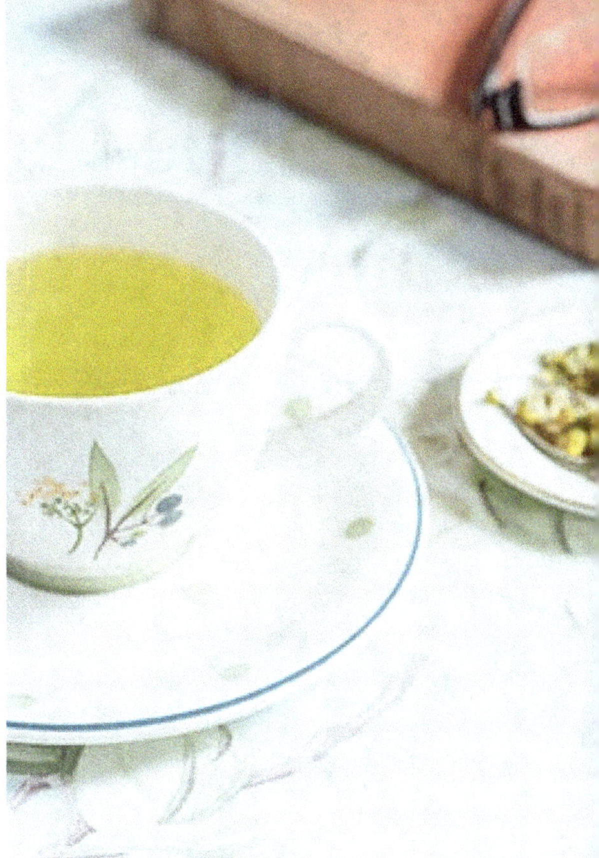

Ingredients :

- 2 tsp dried camomile flowers
- pinch dried lavender, optional
- 2 tsp runny honey

Our Most Popular Alternative

- Honey chicken

Method :

1. Put the camomile and lavender into the teapot and fill up the pot with water that has boiled but been left to stand for 1 min.

Camomile tea with honey

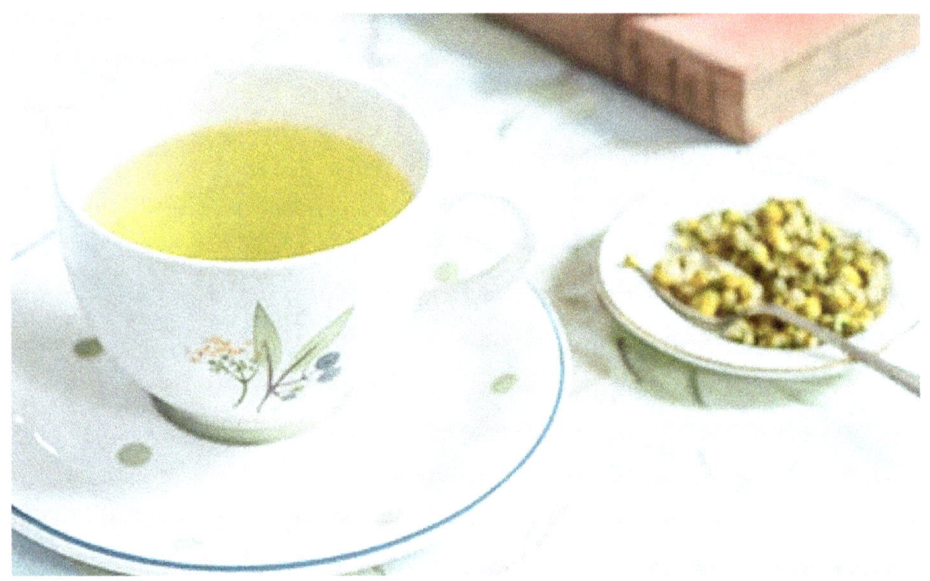

Method :

 Leave the flowers to infuse for 2-3 mins, stir in the honey then strain in to cups to serve.

Wind down in the evening with a calming cup of camomile tea with honey. Use dried camomile flowers with aromatic lavender to make this wonderfully relaxing herbal tea. The petals release a gentle, slightly sweet flavour with notes of honey and apple. A deliciously soothing mix.

GREEN TEA WITH GRAPEFRUIT

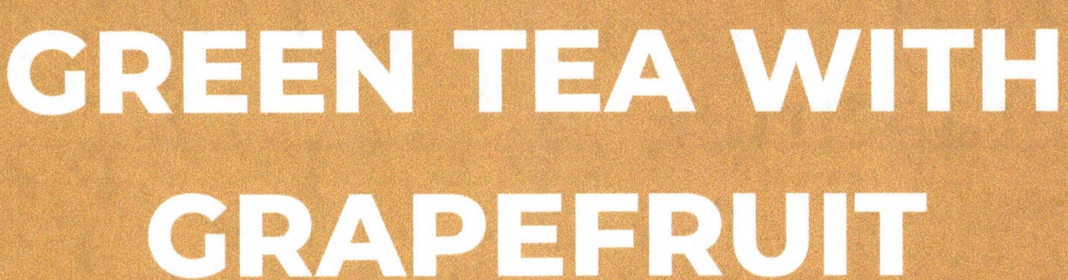

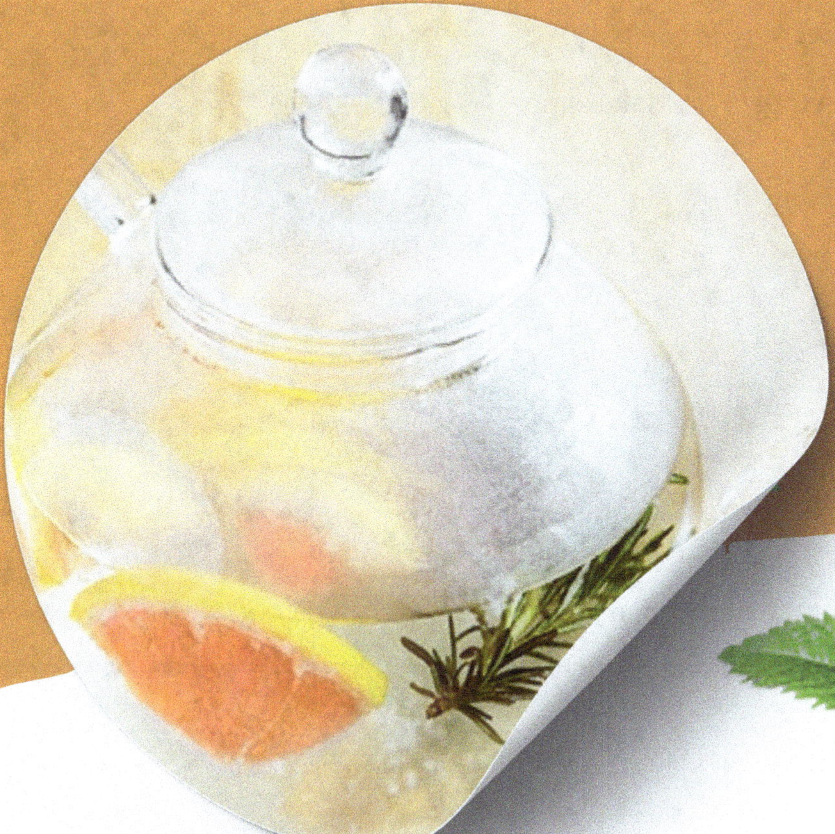

Combine green whole leaf tea with grapefruit slices and a sprig of rosemary to make this refreshing tea blend. Sweeten with honey or agave syrup to taste

Green tea with grapefruit

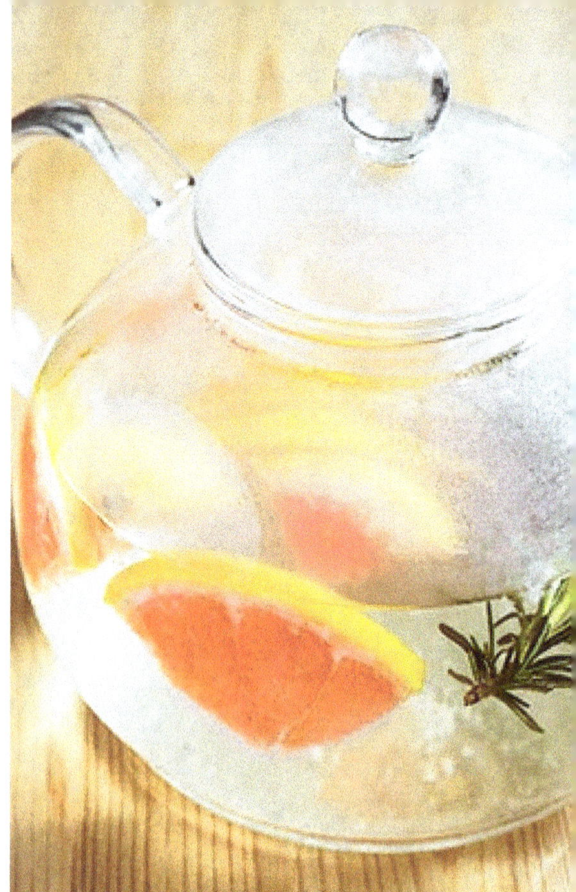

Prep Time : 5 mins

Level : Easy

Servings : Makes one 500-600ml pot (serves 1-2)

Ingredients :

- 2 tsp green whole leaf tea
- ¼ grapefruit, sliced
- sprig of rosemary
- honey or agave syrup to taste

Method :

1. Pour 150ml cold water into a large heatproof jug then top up with 450ml boiling water. Add the tea leaves and leave to steep for 2 mins.

Green tea with grapefruit

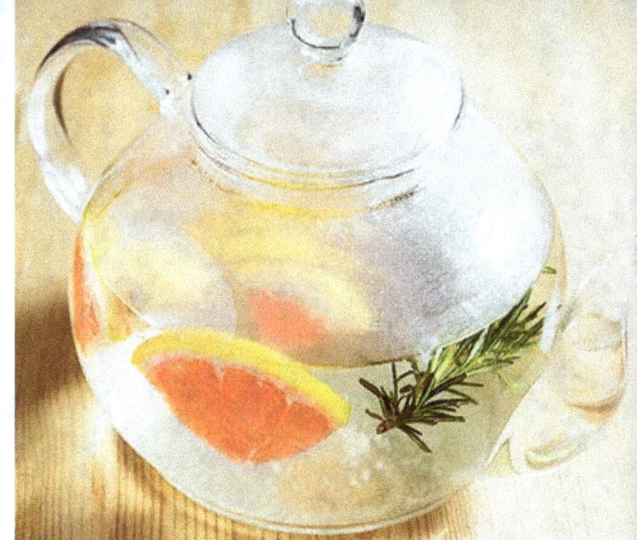

Procedure :

2   Meanwhile, fill your teapot with boiling water to warm it. Once the tea has steeped, pour away the water in the teapot then add the grapefruit and rosemary. Strain the green tea into the teapot, leaving the tea leaves behind. Don't throw the leaves away – you can re-brew them again for another pot that same day. (For the second brew, make sure you let the mixture steep for 3-4 mins.)

3   Let the grapefruit and rosemary infuse for a few moments, then serve. Add honey or agave syrup to sweeten if you like.

Try our zingy green tea with grapefruit for a tasty twist on your classic herbal brew. Add a sprig of rosemary for an aromatic edge, or if you need a touch of sweetness, add some honey or agave syrup. To brew a second pot, leave the mixture to steep for 3-4 minutes rather than two to get the full flavour.

OREGANO TEA

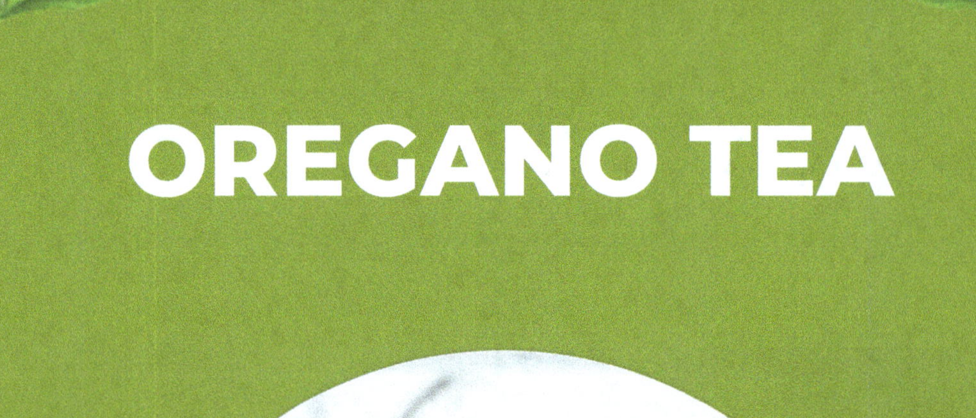

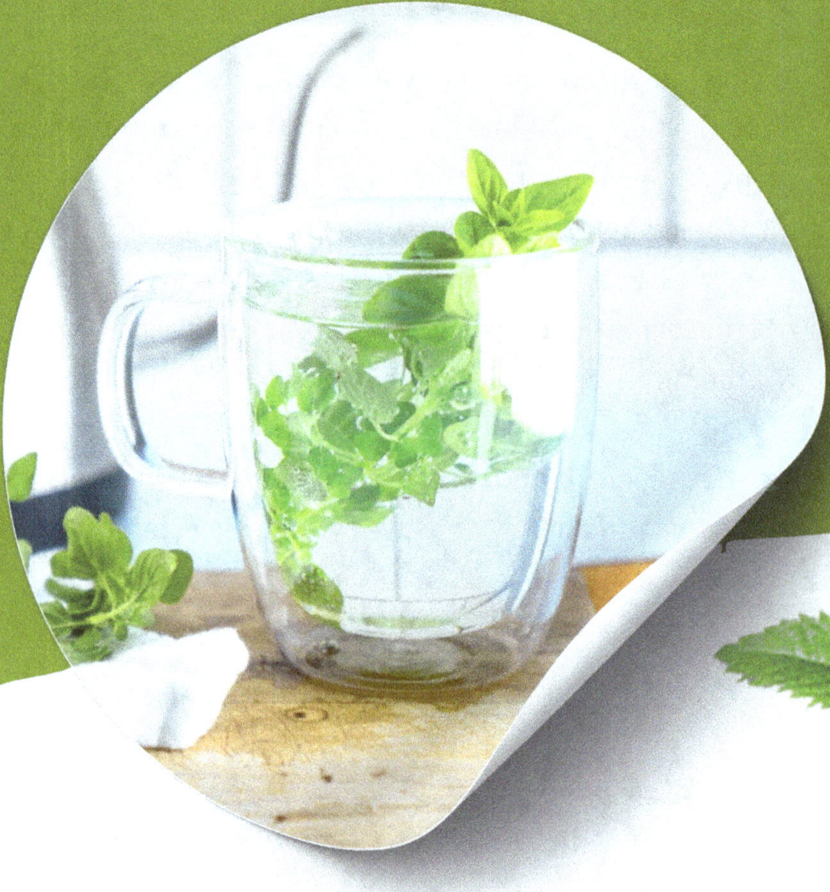

Here's how to make oregano tea, a restorative herbal tea made with just boiling water and fresh oregano! The perfect way to use this fresh herb.

Oregano tea

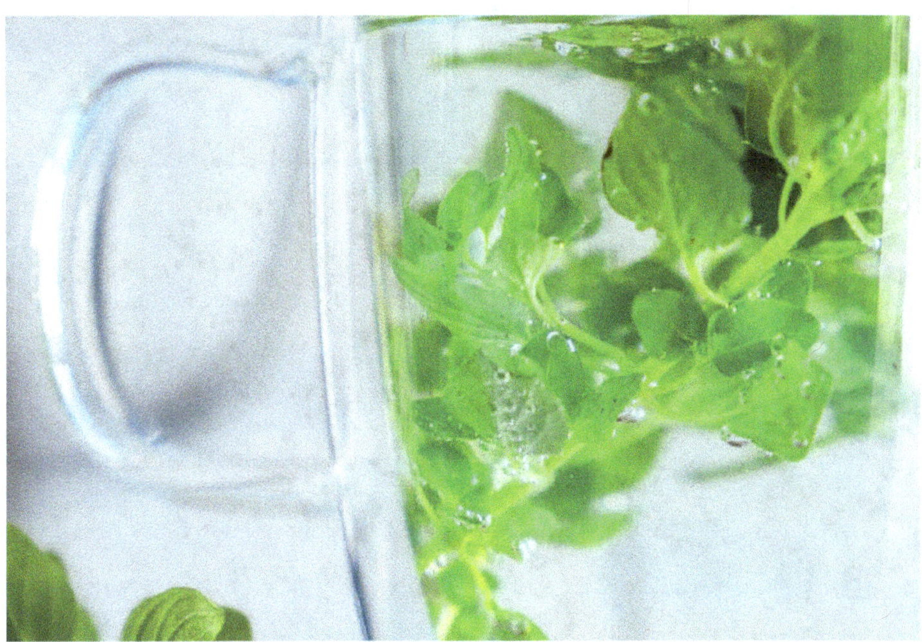

Prep Time : 5 mins

Level : Easy

Servings : 1 drink

Ingredients :

- 2 large leafy fresh oregano sprigs (see photo)
- Boiling water

Method :

1. Bring the water to a boil.

2. Wash the oregano thoroughly.

Oregano tea

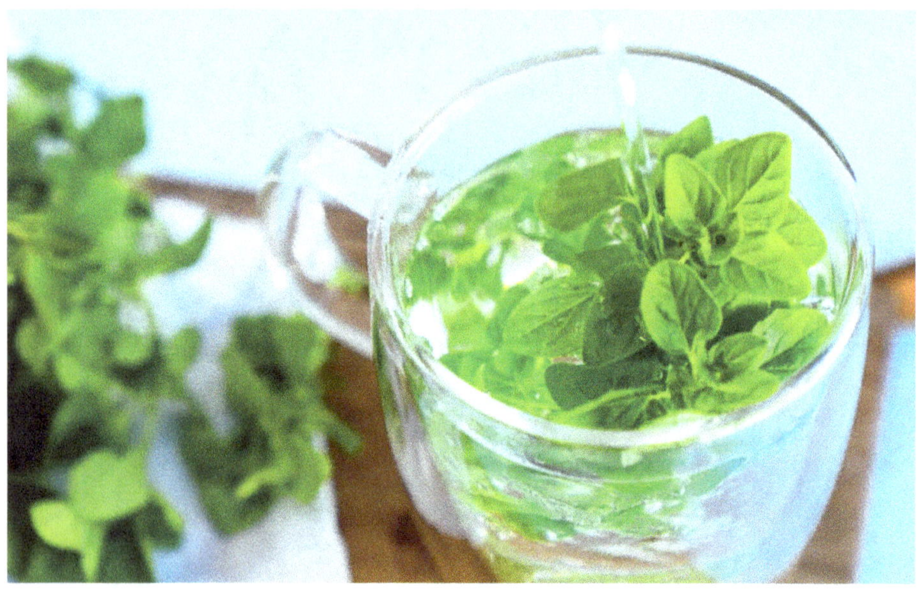

Method :

3. Place the oregano sprigs in a mug, and pour over the boiling water. Allow the herbs to steep for 5 minutes. Remove the oregano and enjoy. (Alternate method: If you prefer, you can also chop the oregano leaves and place them in a tea strainer before steeping.)

Fresh oregano transforms in 5 minutes into an earthy, fresh herbal tea that's positively restorative! All you need is a few sprigs and boiling water! While oregano is best known for flavoring Italian recipes, its flavor lends intrigue to tea. This recipe is best in the summer when you've got fresh herbs growing in your garden or in pots. .

ROOIBOS & PEAR TEA

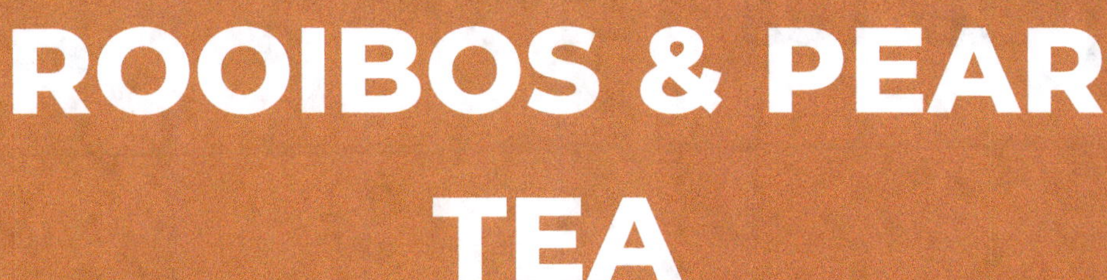

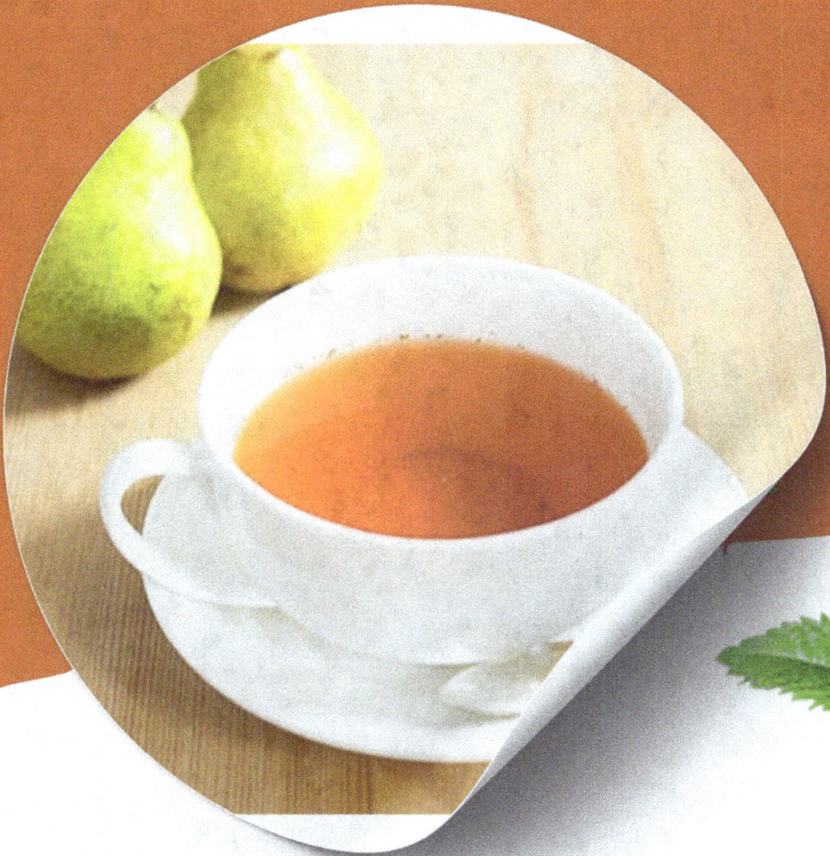

Add a twist to rooibos tea with the addition of fresh pear and a fragrant cinnamon stick. Garnish with extra pear slices to impress guests at an afternoon tea

Rooibos & pear tea

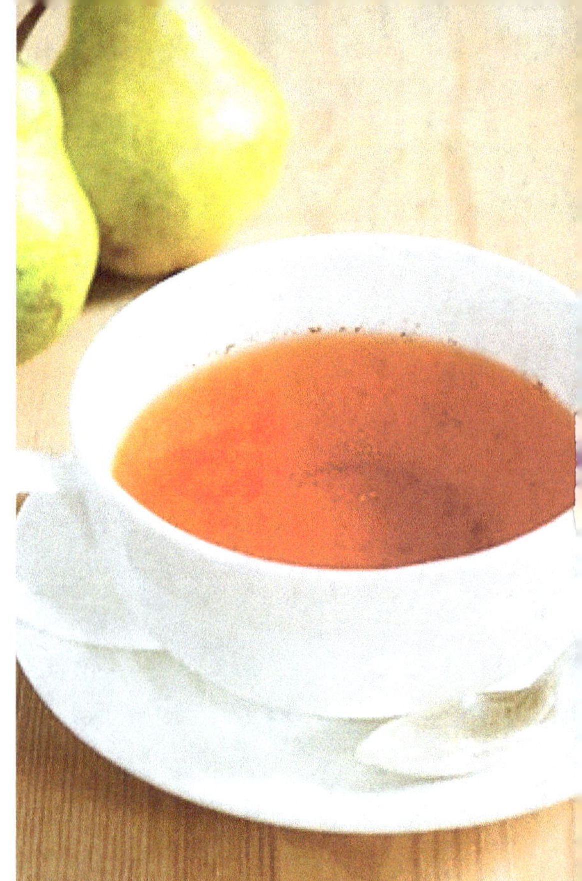

Prep Time : 5 mins

Level : Easy

Servings : Makes one 500-600ml pot (serves 1-2)

Ingredients :

- 1 ripe pear, sliced
- ½ a cinnamon stick
- 2 tsp rooibos leaf tea

Our Most Popular Alternative

- Pear crumble

Method :

1. Put the pear slices into a large saucepan and add 600ml water and the piece of cinnamon stick – keep a slice or 2 of pear back to use as decoration later if you like. Bring to a simmer, then cook the pear slices for 5-6 mins or until softening.

Rooibos & pear tea

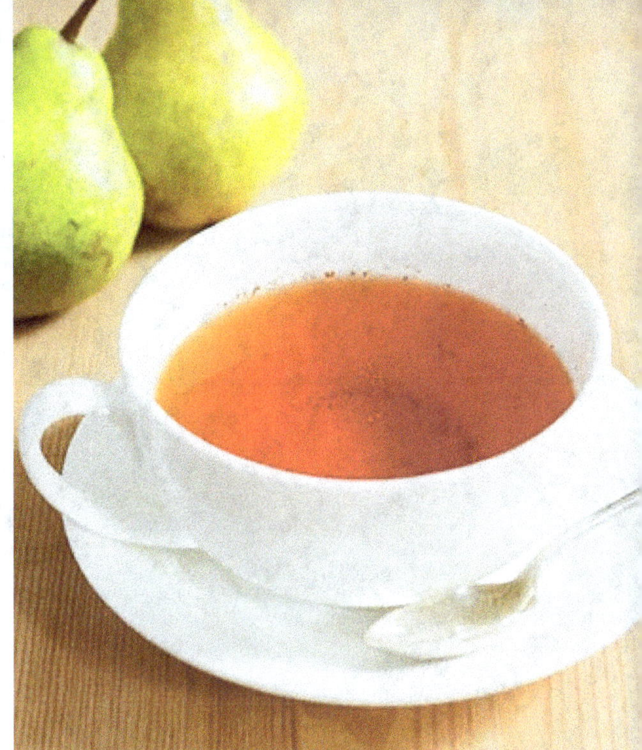

Method :

2 Take the pan off the heat and add the rooibos tea.

3 Let the mixture steep for 2-3 mins then strain into a warm teapot to serve, garnished with extra pear slices if you like.

Our rust-red, caffeine-free rooibos & pear tea with sweet-smelling cinnamon and delicate pear is an impressive cuppa, but it's deceptively simple to make. Garnish with extra slices of pear to wow your guests at your next afternoon tea. The robust, slightly sweet flavour of the tea leaves pairs perfectly with light and fruity pear and full-bodied cinnamon spice.

CINNAMON TEA

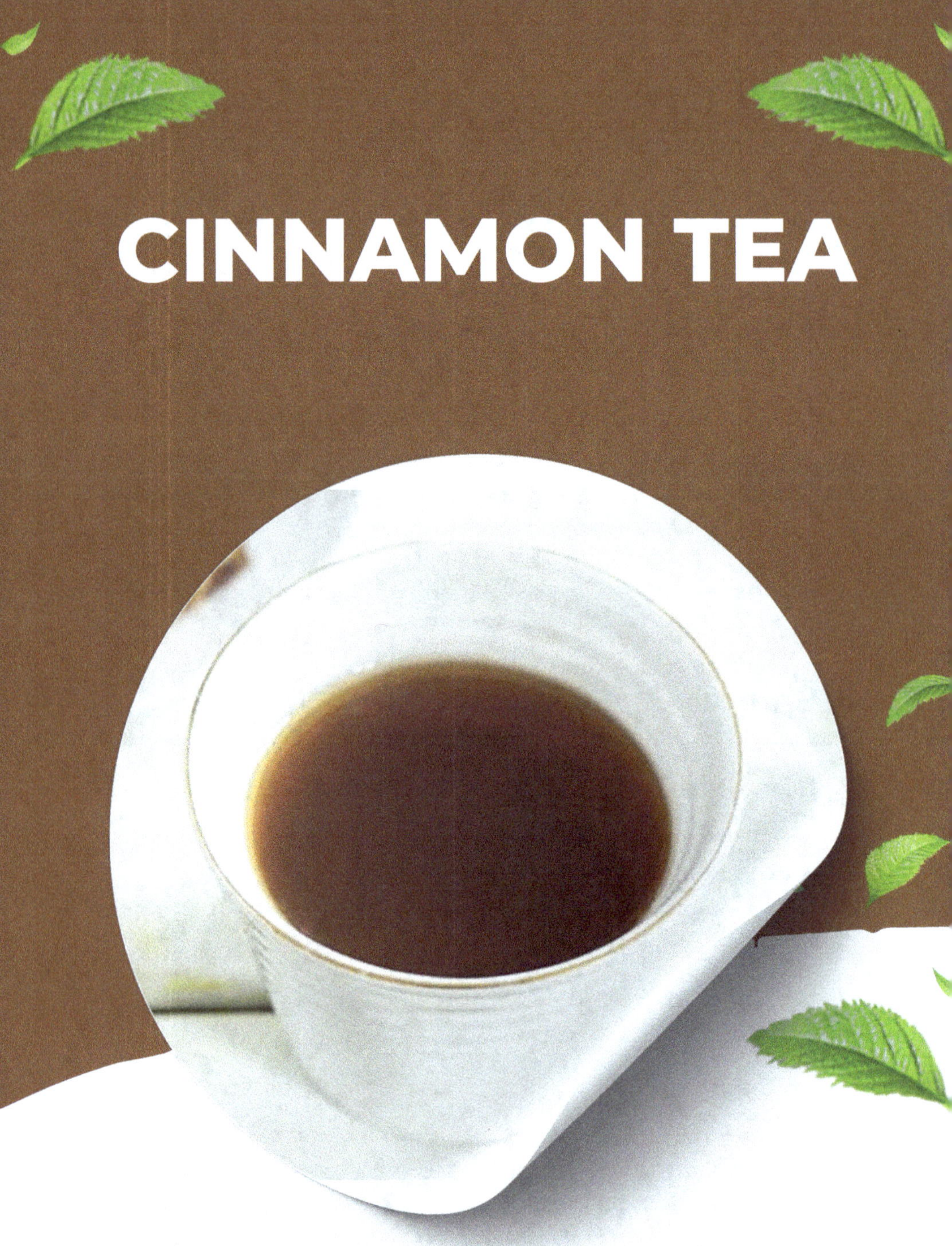

Add a cinnamon stick to an assam leaf tea to make this warming cinnamon-spiced brew that's great on cold days. Sweeten with a dollop of honey to taste

Cinnamon tea

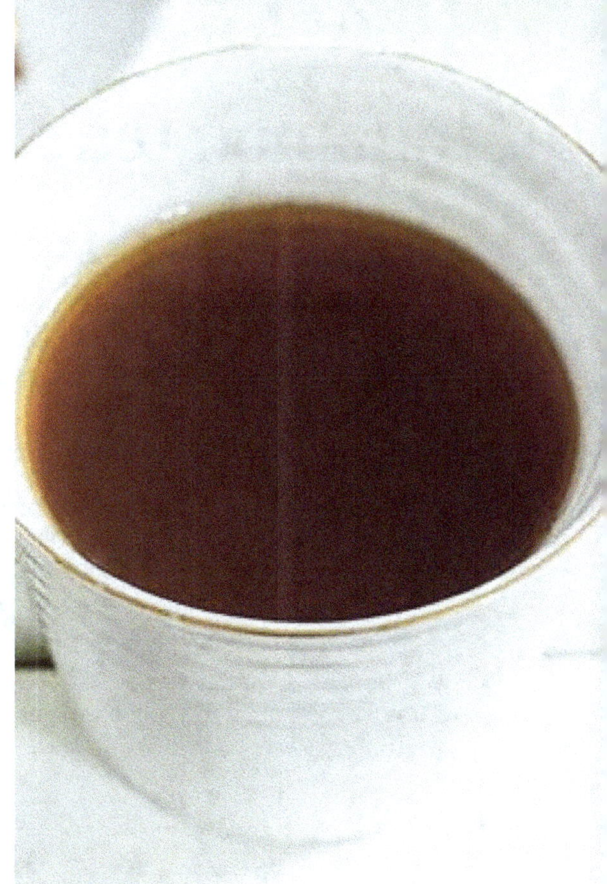

Prep Time : 5 mins

Level : Easy

Servings : Makes one 500-600ml pot (serves 1-2)

Ingredients :

- 1 cinnamon stick
- 2 tsp assam leaf tea
- honey to taste

Our Most Popular Alternative

- Easy carrot cake

Method :

1 Fill a large teapot with just-boiled water to warm it and set aside. Heat 600ml water in a pan with a cinnamon stick until boiling.

Cinnamon tea

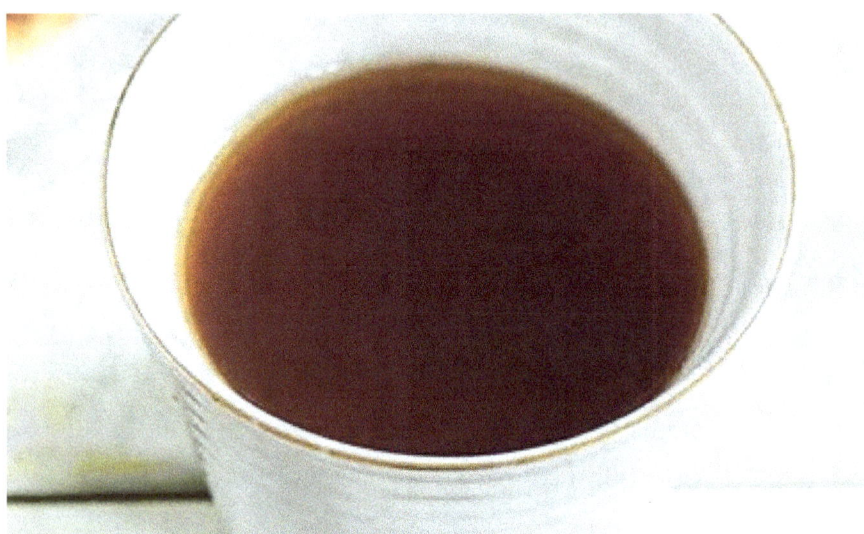

Method :

2. Turn off the heat, add the assam tea leaves to the hot cinnamon water and leave to steep for 1-2 mins. Remove the cinnamon stick.

3. Empty the teapot and strain the tea into it. Serve with honey to sweeten to taste.

Enhance your Assam leaf tea experience by introducing a fragrant cinnamon stick, transforming it into a warming cinnamon-spiced brew perfect for chilly days. Sweeten it with a dollop of honey to suit your tastes. Not just a warming drink, cinnamon also helps to defend against infection and protects against cold and flus.

LEMON & GINGER TEA

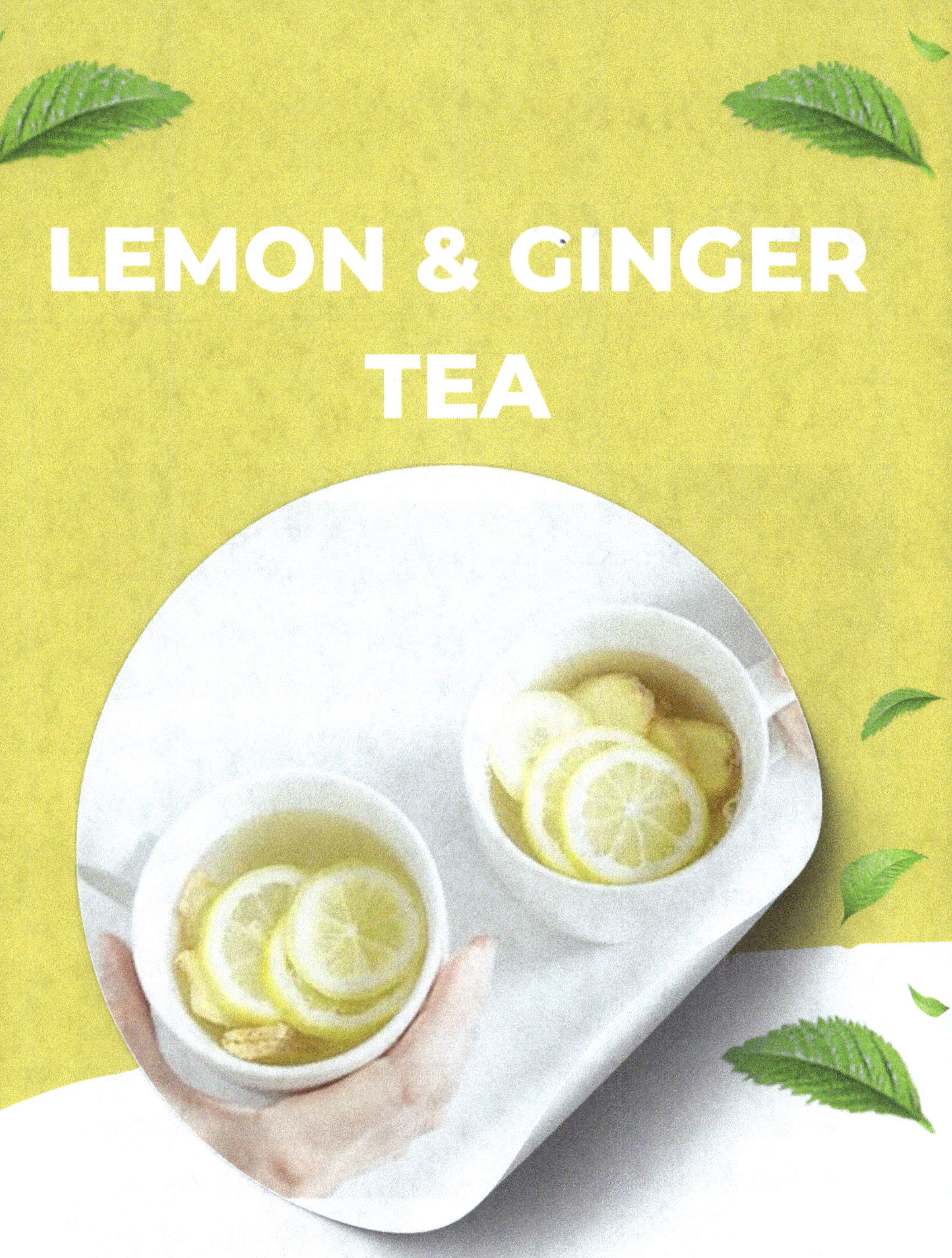

Combine lemon with root ginger to make this refreshing lemon and ginger tea that's a great alternative to caffeinated drinks. Sweeten with honey if you like

Lemon & ginger tea

Prep Time : 5 mins

Level : Easy

Servings : Serves 2

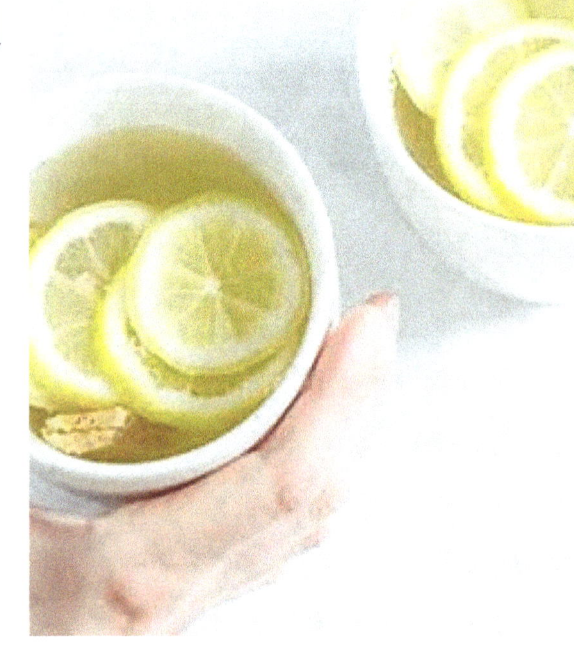

Ingredients :

- 1 lemon
- 2cm piece root ginger, finely sliced
- honey to taste

Our Most Popular Alternative

- Ginger shots

Method :

1. Cut the lemon in half. Squeeze the juice from one half and slice the rest. Divide the lemon juice and slices between 2 mugs, along with the sliced ginger.

Lemon & ginger tea

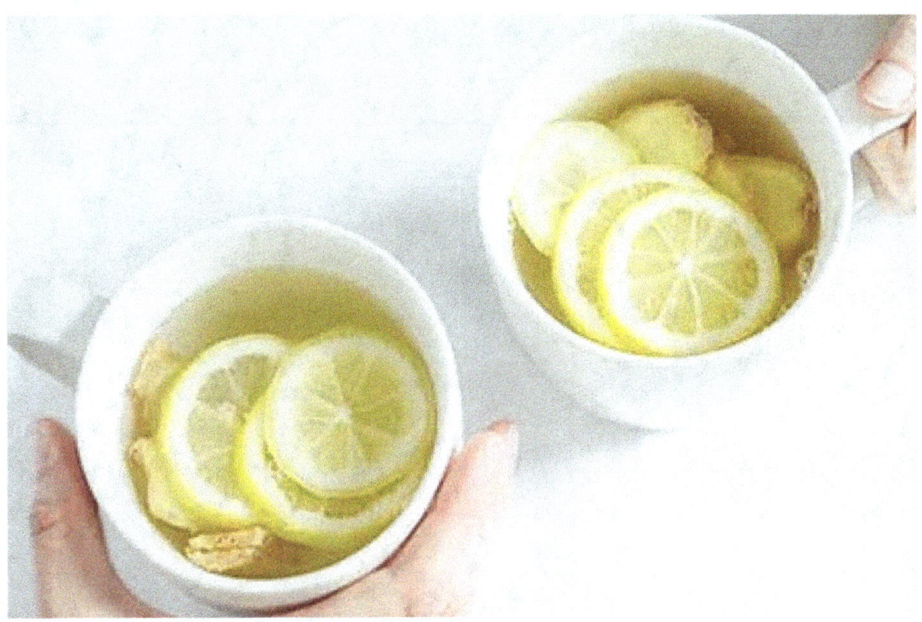

Method :

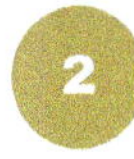 2 Fill the mugs with boiling water and leave to steep for 3 mins or until cool enough to sip. Sweeten with honey if you like.

Three key ingredients make up our lemon & ginger tea; it makes a punchy alternative to caffeinated drinks. Use fine slices of fresh root ginger and segments of lemon to create an invigorating mugful of flavour. Feeling a little under the weather or in need of a warming dose of vitamin C? Look no further. This is also the ideal tipple to soothe a sore throat. Sweeten it up with a squeeze of honey if needed.

LAVENDER TEA

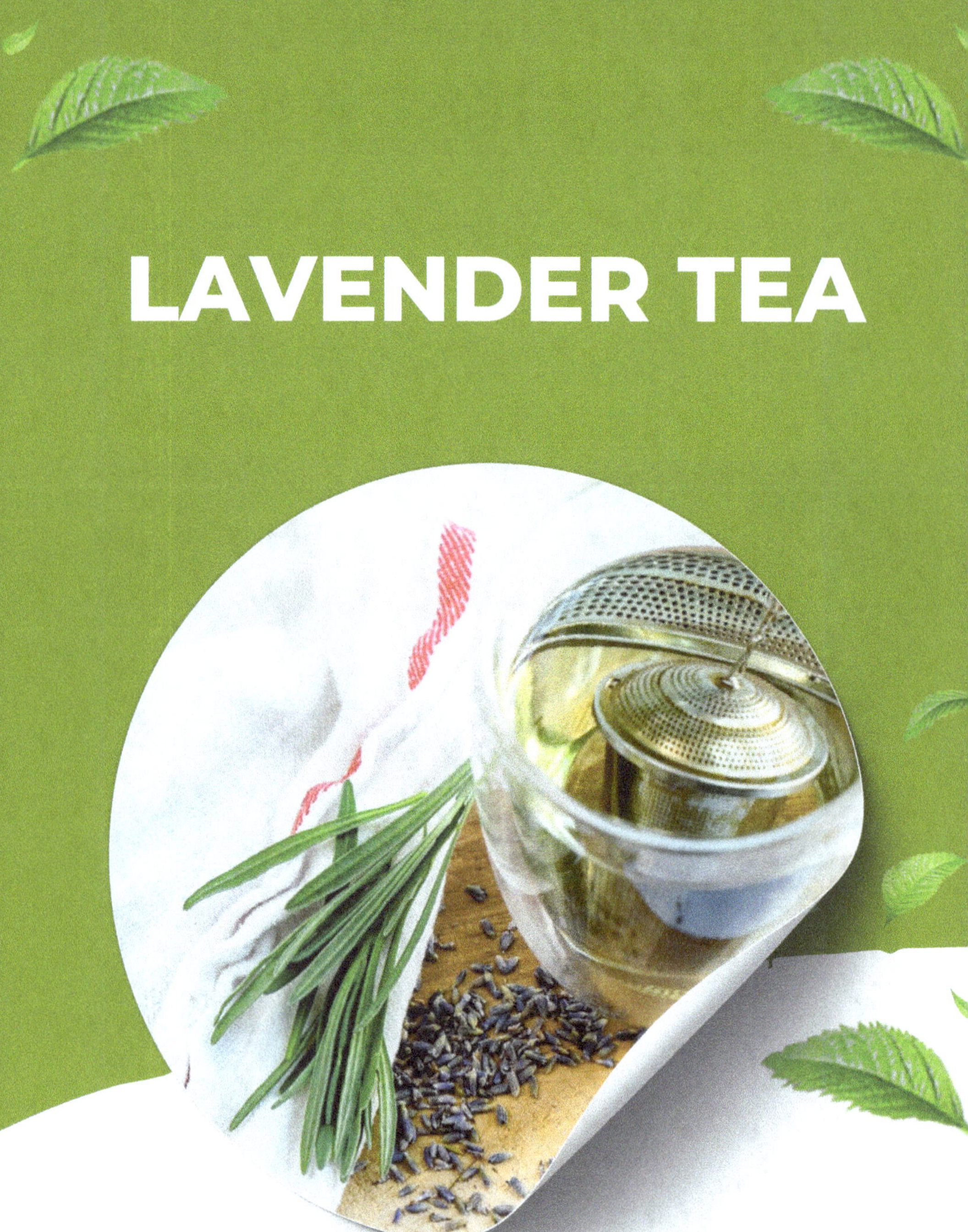

Here's how to make oregano tea, a restorative herbal tea made with just boiling water and fresh oregano! The perfect way to use this fresh herb.

Lavender Tea

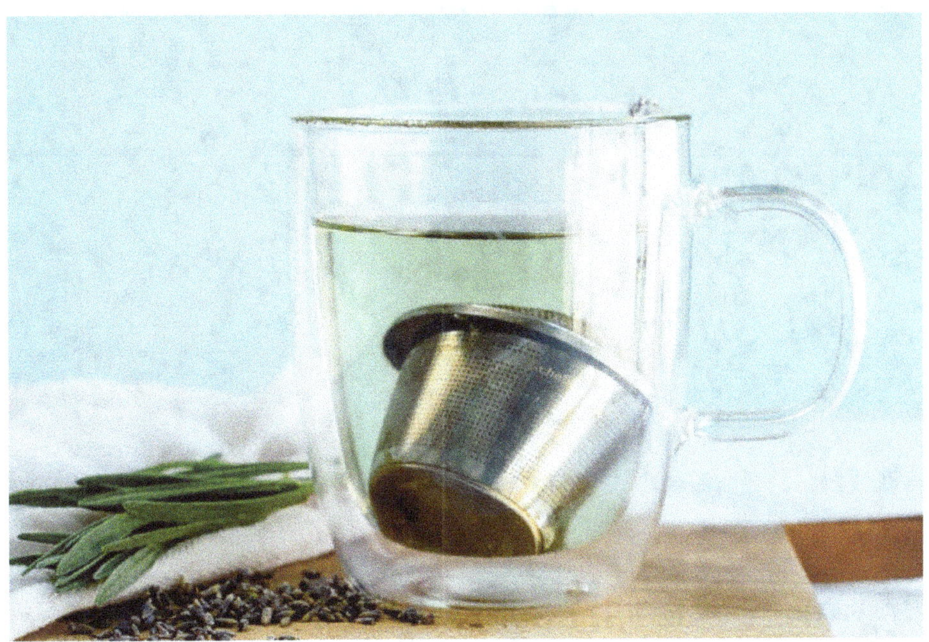

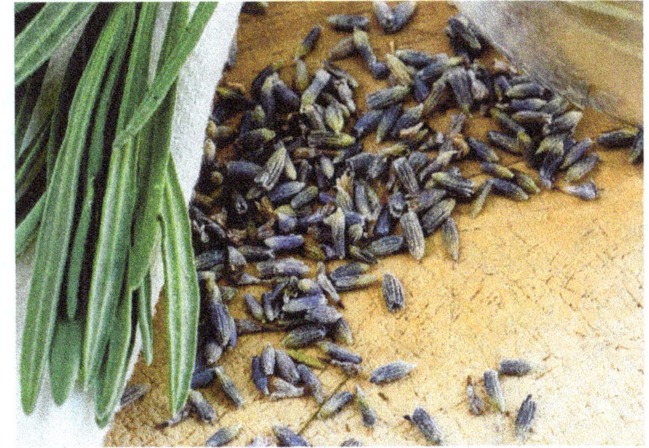

Prep Time : 5 mins

Level : Easy

Servings : 1 drink

Ingredients :

- 1 ¼ cups (10 ounces) boiling water
- 2 teaspoons lavender buds, dried or fresh
- 1 teaspoon honey (or maple syrup or agave syrup)

Lavender Tea

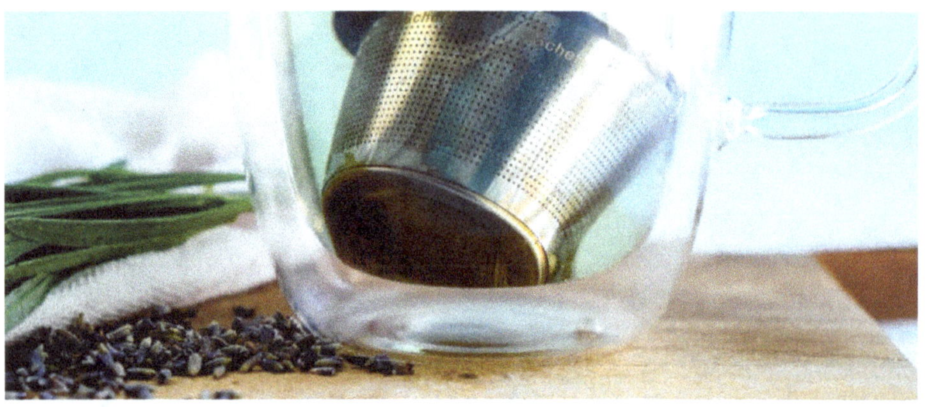

Method :

1. Bring the water to a boil.

2. Place the lavender buds in a tea strainer or tea ball. When the water is hot, steep in a tea strainer in the water for 5 minutes.

3. Remove the tea strainer and stir in the honey. Enjoy immediately!

Lavender herbal tea is uniquely delicious! Tea made with lavender blossoms has a subtle floral undertone. Sweetened with honey it's a delightfully soothing cup. It has some potential health benefits, too. Here's how to make it!

JASMINE & GINGER TEA

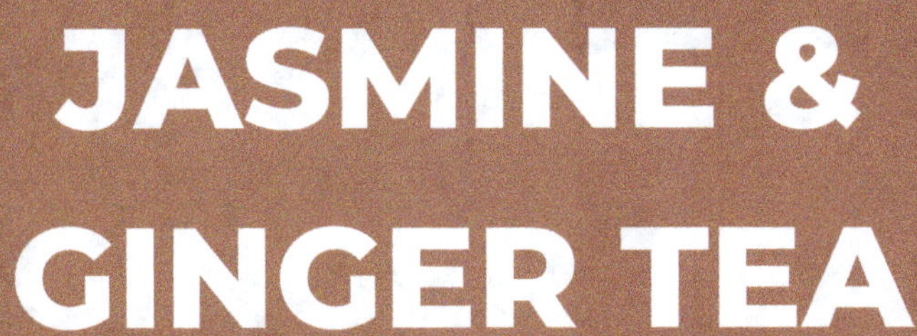

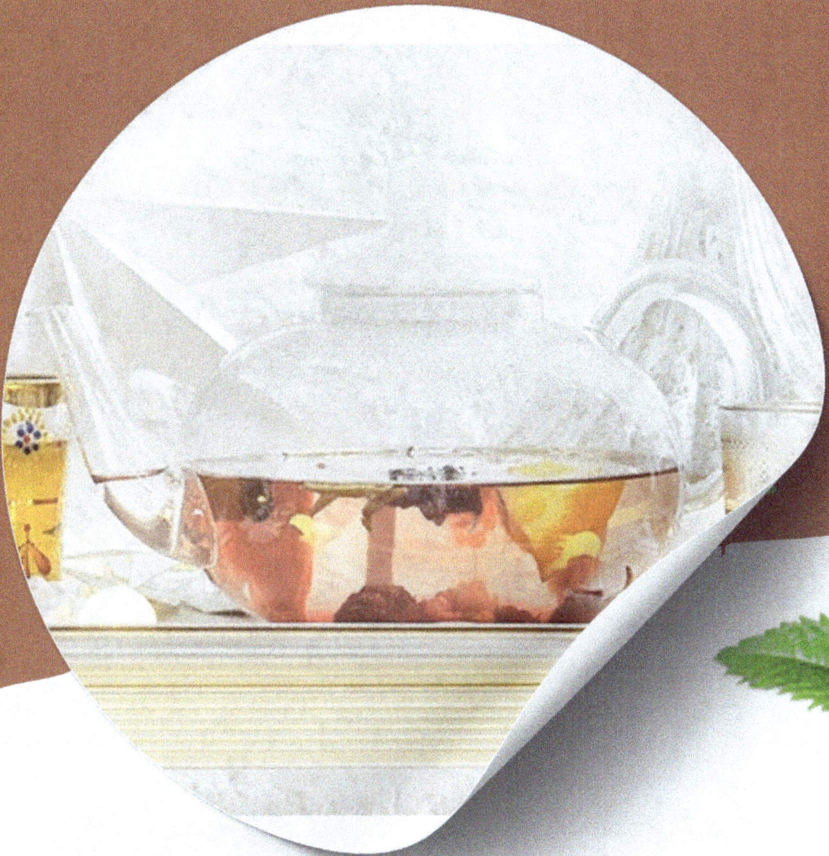

Enjoy a warming pot of jasmine tea with chai spices including cinnamon, star anise, cloves and ginger. The addition of orange and berries adds a fruity tang

Jasmine & ginger tea

Cook Time : 10 mins

Level : Easy

Servings : Serves 2

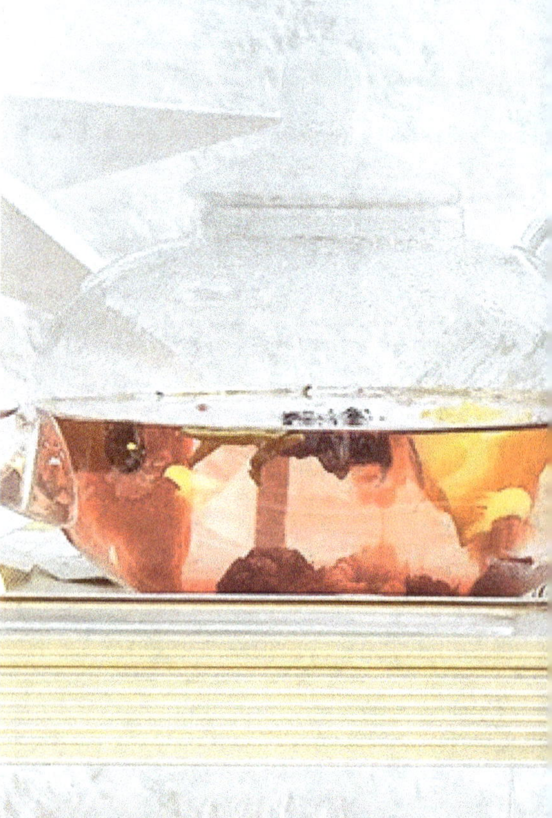

Ingredients :

- 1 tbsp loose leaf jasmine tea
- a handful of frozen berries
- 1 small cinnamon stick
- 1 star anise
- 2 cloves
- a slice of ginger
- a wedge of orange
- 1l water

Method :

1. Put the jasmine tea and frozen berries into a large teapot. Add the cinnamon stick, star anise, cloves, ginger and orange. Fill the teapot with up to 1 litre water.

Jasmine & ginger tea

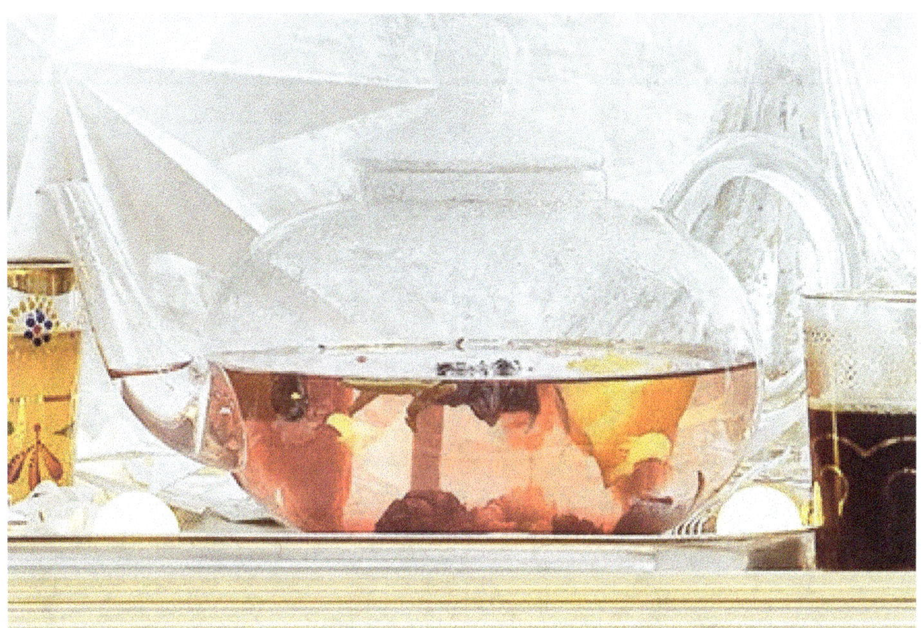

Method :

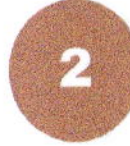 Let it steep for 3-4 mins, then strain into teacups to serve.

Pack in plenty of spice with our jasmine & ginger tea. Enjoy a cup with chai spices including cinnamon, star anise, cloves and ginger. Try adding a wedge of orange or clementine and a handful of frozen berries for a fruity tang. Our simple recipe makes enough for four people, so it's perfect for an impromptu gathering with friends.

MINT & MANGO ICED GREEN TEA

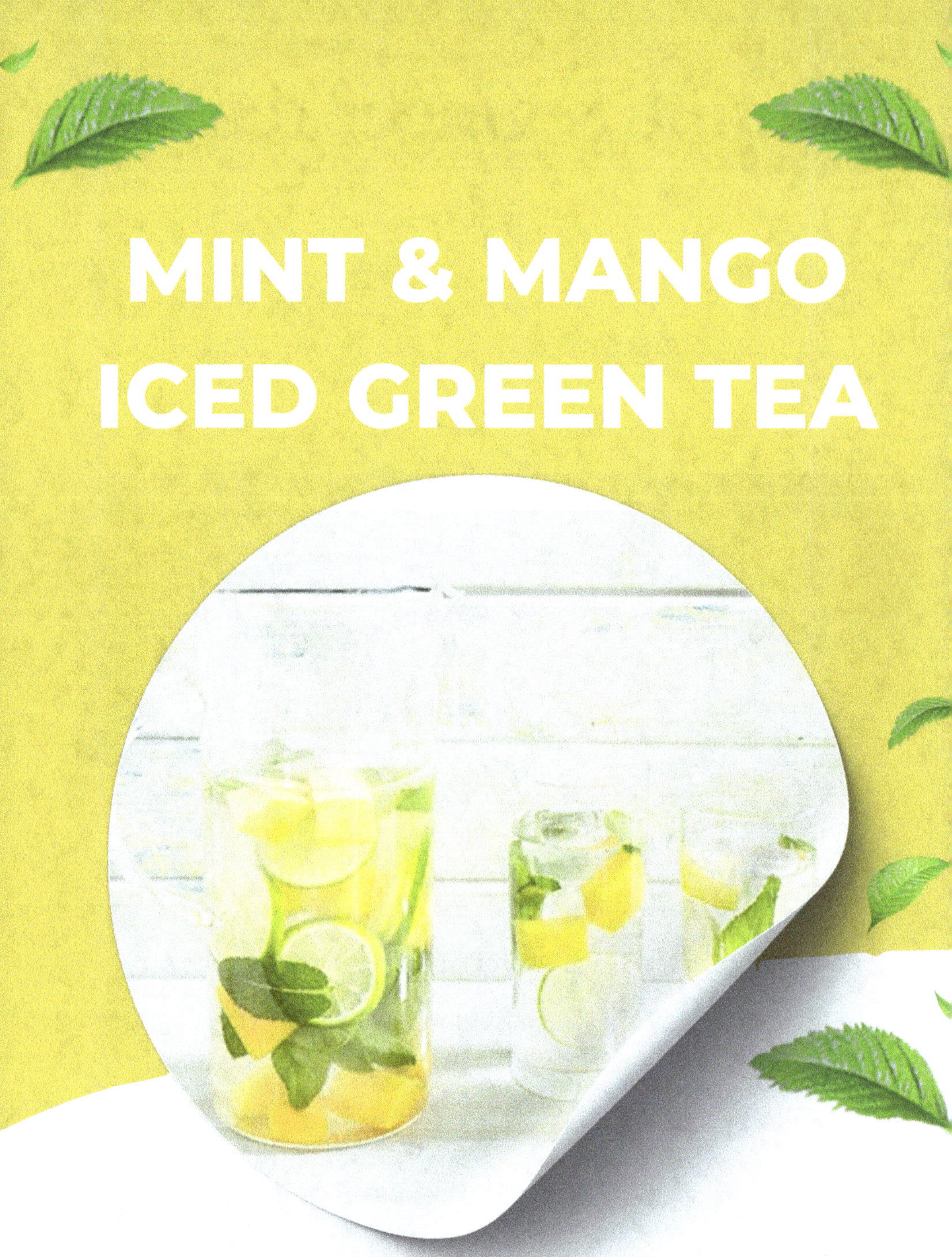

Blend the flavour of green tea with mango, fresh mint, lime and ice to make this iced tea. It makes a wonderfully refreshing summer drink at any time of day

Mint & mango iced green tea

Cook Time : 10 mins

Level : Easy

Servings : Serves 4 - 6

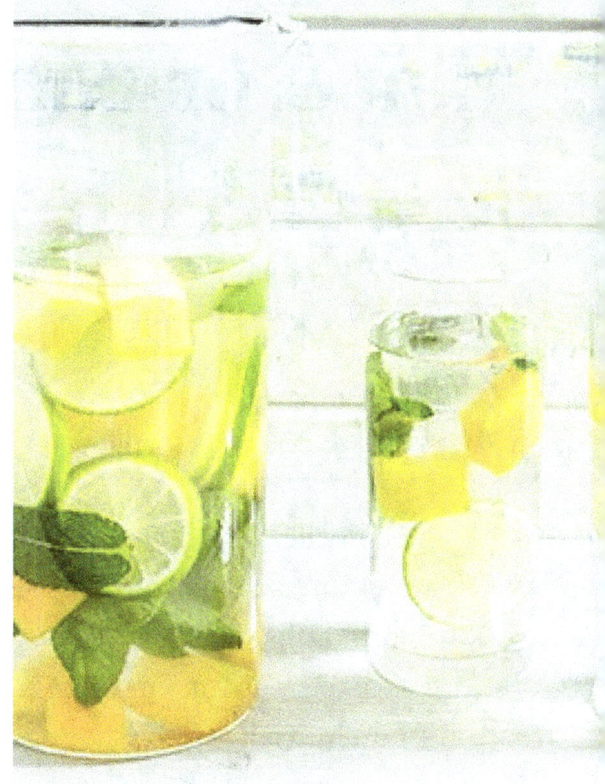

Ingredients :

- 1 mango, peeled, stoned and chopped
- 100g granulated sugar
- 4 tsp green tea leaves
- small bunch fresh mint
- 1 lime, sliced
- ice

Method :

1. Put half the mango in a saucepan with the sugar and 100ml water. Cook for 8-10 mins then strain through a sieve and leave the liquid to cool.

Mint & mango iced green tea

Method :

2. Meanwhile, pour 500ml boiling water into a large heatproof jug and add the green tea leaves. Leave to steep for 5 mins, then strain into a large glass jug and add 300ml cold water. Leave to cool completely then put into the fridge to chill.

3. Once cold, add the strained mango syrup to the chilled tea, along with the rest of the chopped mango, fresh mint and the lime slices. Fill up the jug with ice, stir gently and serve.

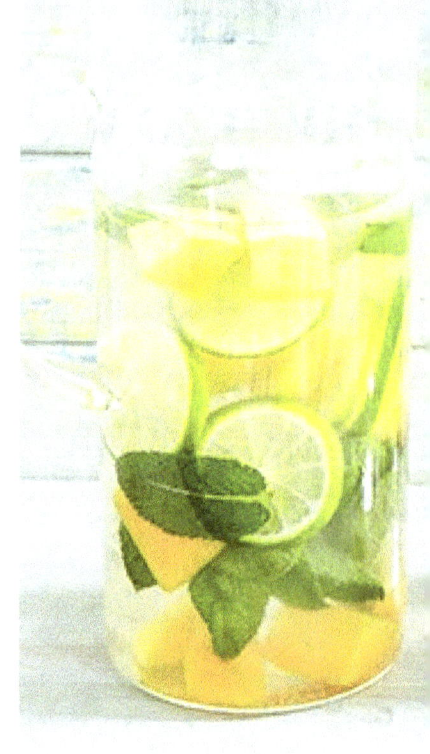

Cool down on a piping hot afternoon with our summery blend of mint & mango iced green tea. Mix up a pitcher for a crowd, then chill in the fridge until needed. Once it's cold, add the mango syrup, mint and chopped fruit for a satisfying refreshment. Try topping up with a dash of sparkling water for an easy mocktail you can make in just 15 minutes.

MATCHA WITH VANILLA

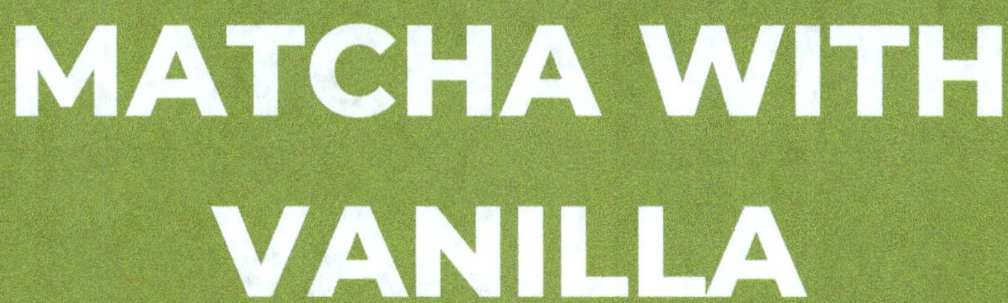

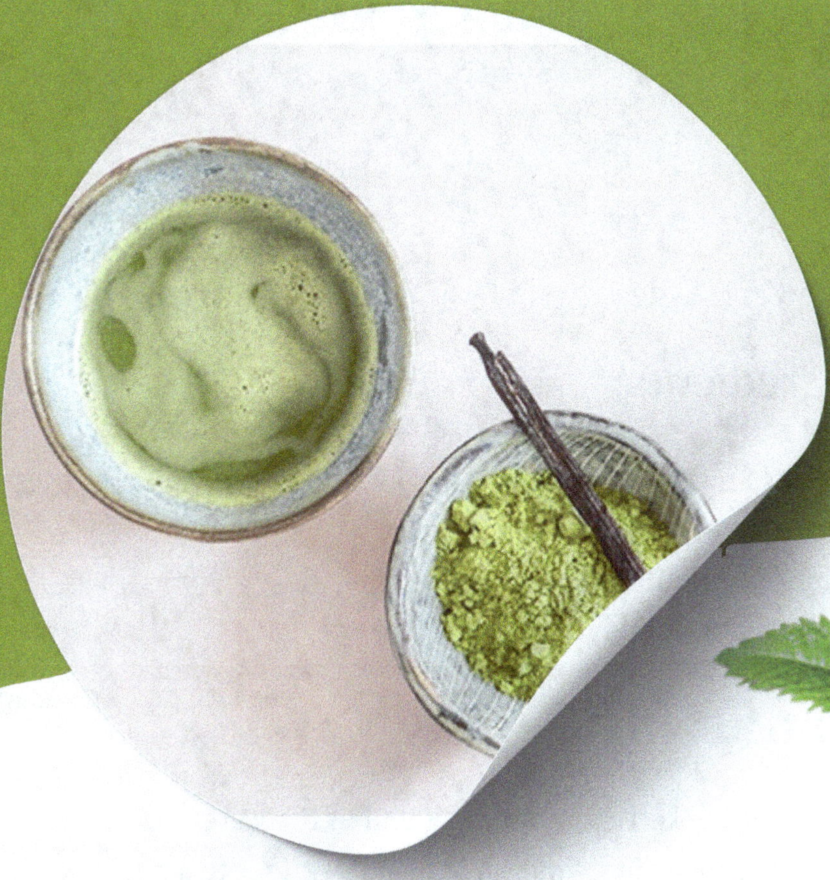

Swap your regular tea or coffee for this delicious Japanese-style green matcha and vanilla tea. It's simple to make at home and takes just five minutes

Matcha with vanilla

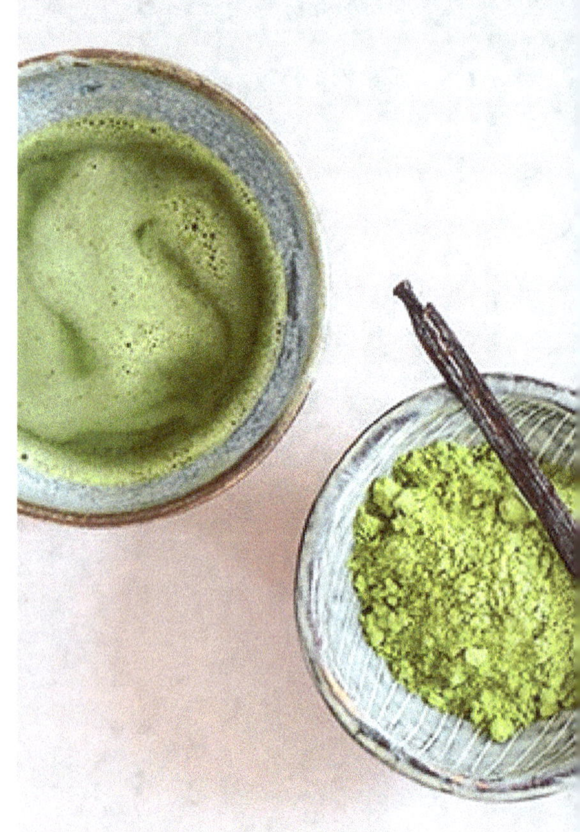

Prep Time : 5 mins

Level : Easy

Servings : Serves 1

Ingredients :

- ½ tsp matcha powder
- seeds from half a vanilla pod

Our Most Popular Alternative

- Ultimate vanilla ice cream

Method :

1. Boil the kettle then pour 100ml of the water into a measuring jug. Pour half the hot water into a small bowl, to warm it, then add the matcha powder and vanilla seeds to the rest of the water in the jug.

Matcha with vanilla

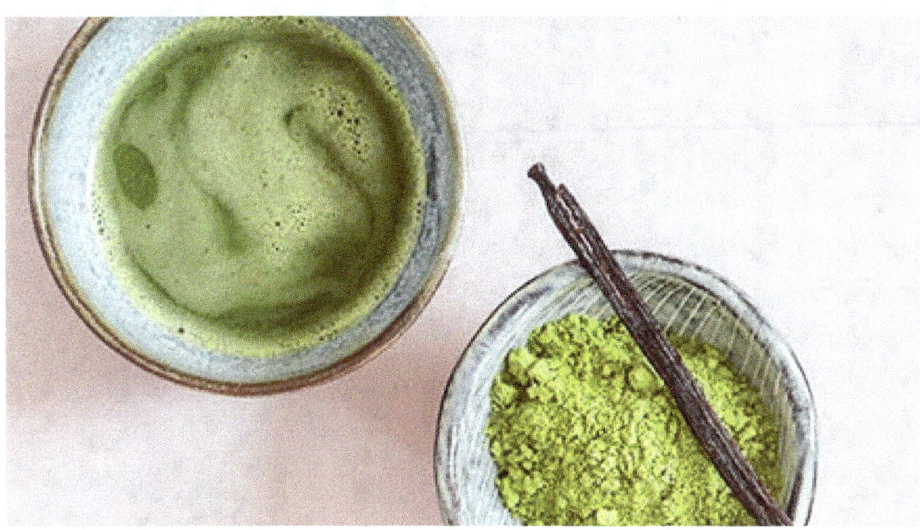

Method :

2. Whisk the mixture with a bamboo match whisk or mini electric whisk until it's smooth, lump-free and slightly bubbly. Discard the water in the warmed tea bowl, then pour in the prepared matcha tea.

Swap your regular cup of coffee for this delicious green matcha with vanilla tea. This easy, Japanese-style drink boasts a rich, complex taste with lingering sweetness, and takes just five minutes to make. Want something with a little more body? Try our foamy, café-style matcha latte.

BLUEBERRY & MINT ICED TEA

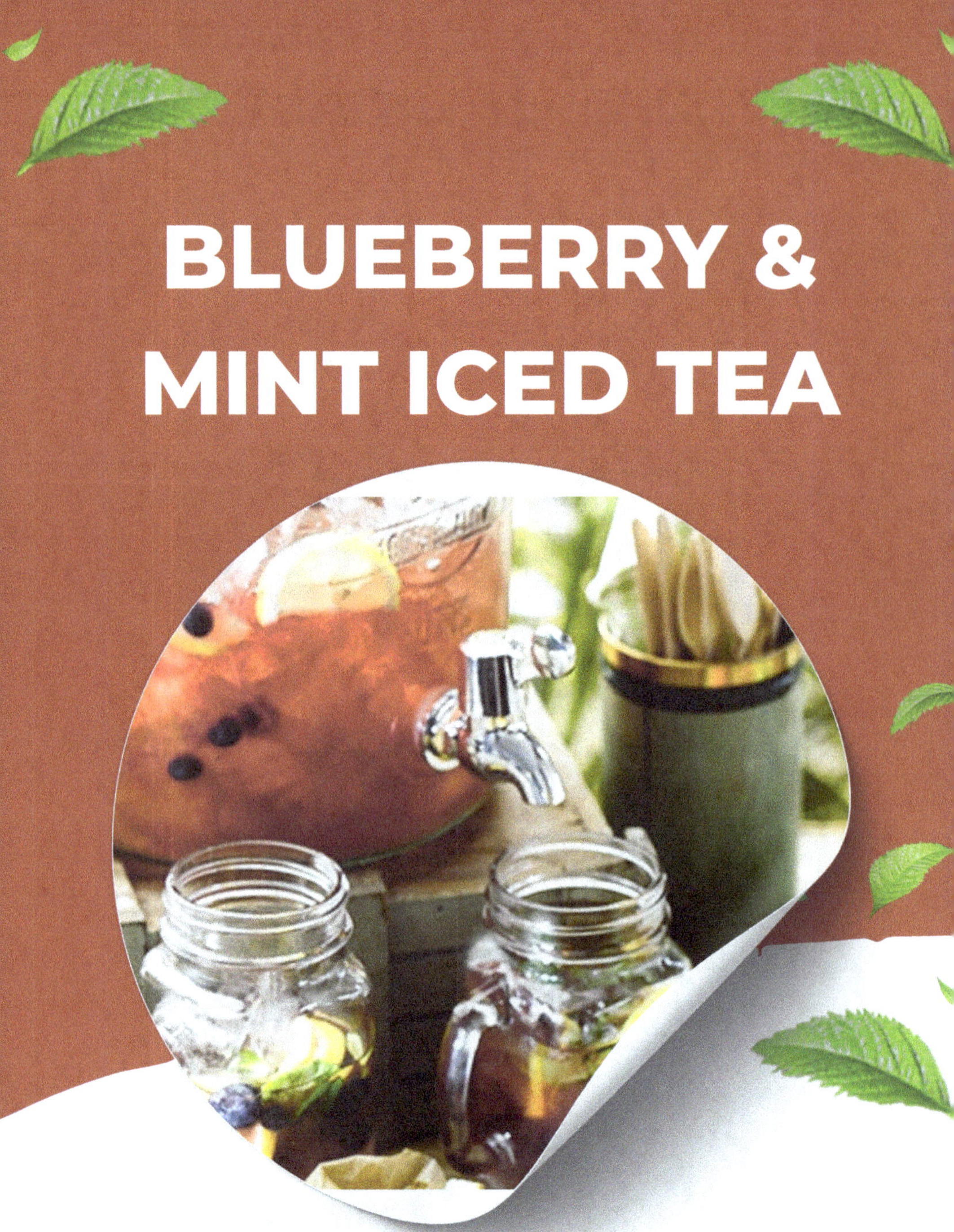

Refreshing and fruity, this delicious drink is guaranteed to please at a family picnic, barbecue or party

Blueberry & mint iced tea

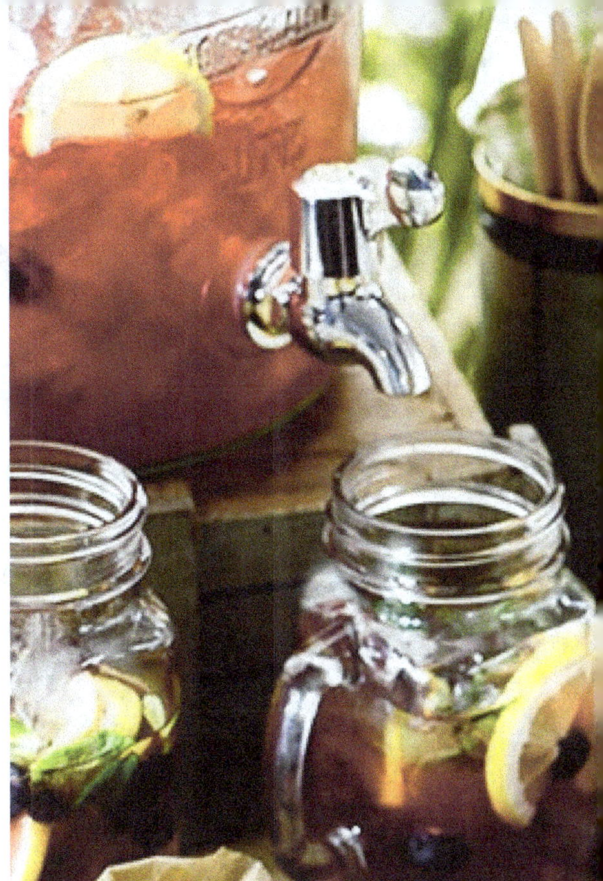

Prep Time : 5 mins

Level : Easy

Servings : Serves 4

Ingredients :

- 5 peppermint tea bags
- 140g blueberries
- 2 tbsp golden caster sugar
- large handful ice
- handful mint leaves
- a few lemon slices

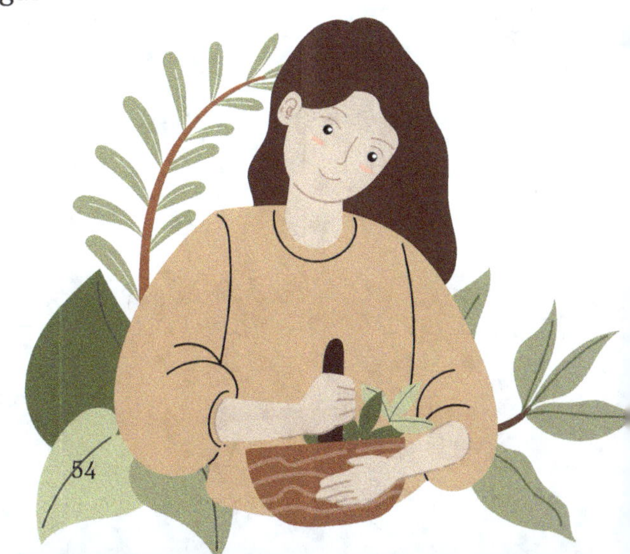

Blueberry & mint iced tea

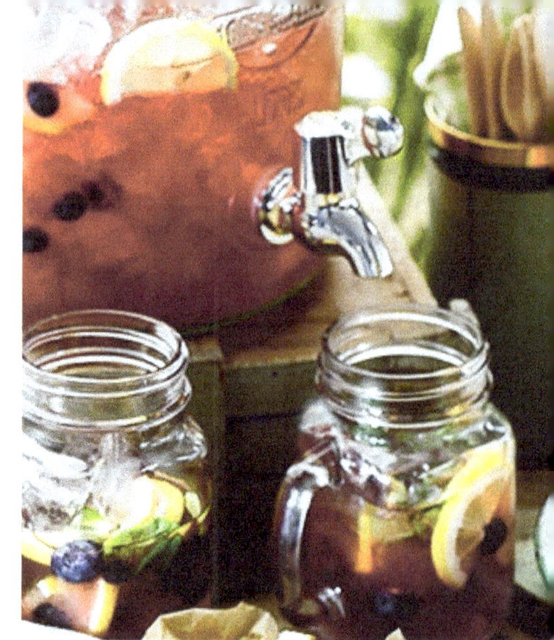

Method :

1. Boil the kettle and put the tea bags in a jug. Pour over 500ml boiling water and leave to steep for 5 mins. Meanwhile, put 100g blueberries in a jug, add the sugar and lightly crush with the end of a rolling pin or a potato masher. Remove the tea bags from the water, pour the tea over the blueberries and top up with another 300ml cold water. Add a large handful of ice to cool quickly, or chill until cold.

2. When you're ready to pack your picnic, pour the iced tea into bottles or flasks. Add a few sprigs of fresh mint, some lemon slices and the remaining blueberries. Seal and store in a cooler bag.

Enjoy this refreshing crowd-pleaser at family picnics, barbecues, or parties. Including nutrient-rich blueberries contributes to your 5-a-day and adds fruity flavours.

CHAI TEA

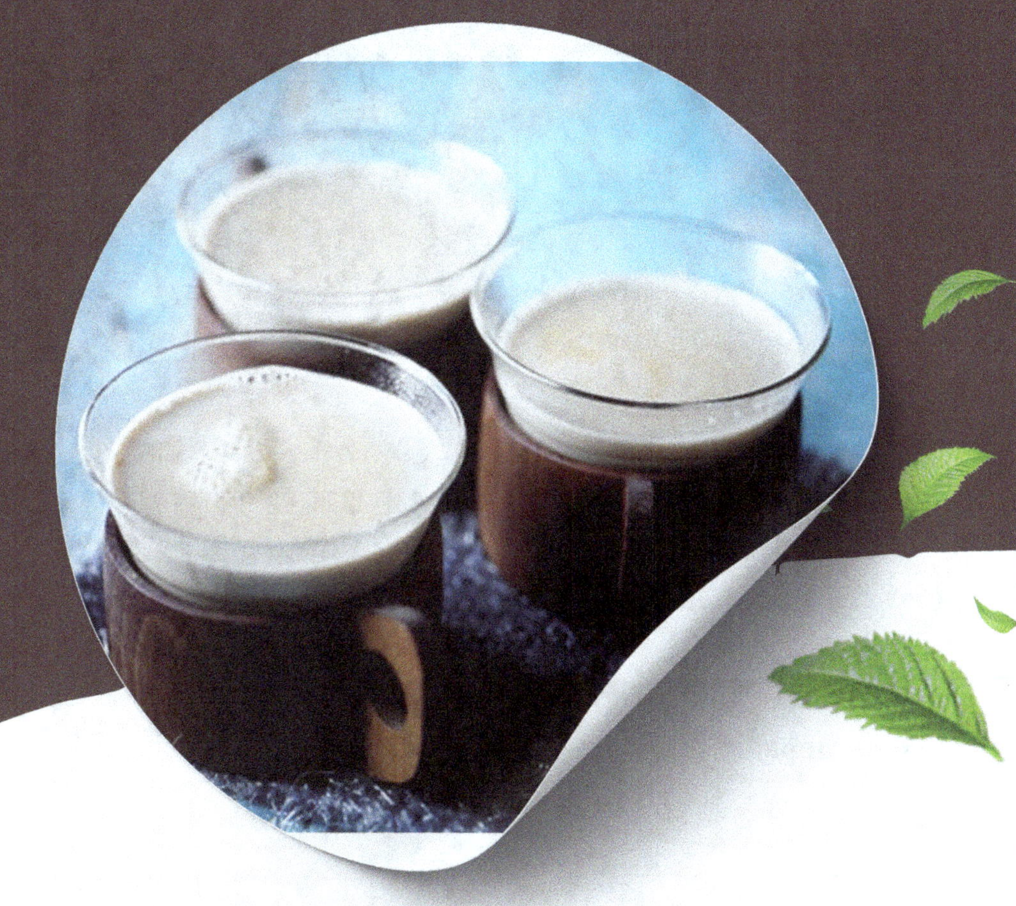

A warming spiced tea, that's the perfect match for our coconut chai traybake. A quick and easy brew that can be made with almond or cow's milk

Chai tea

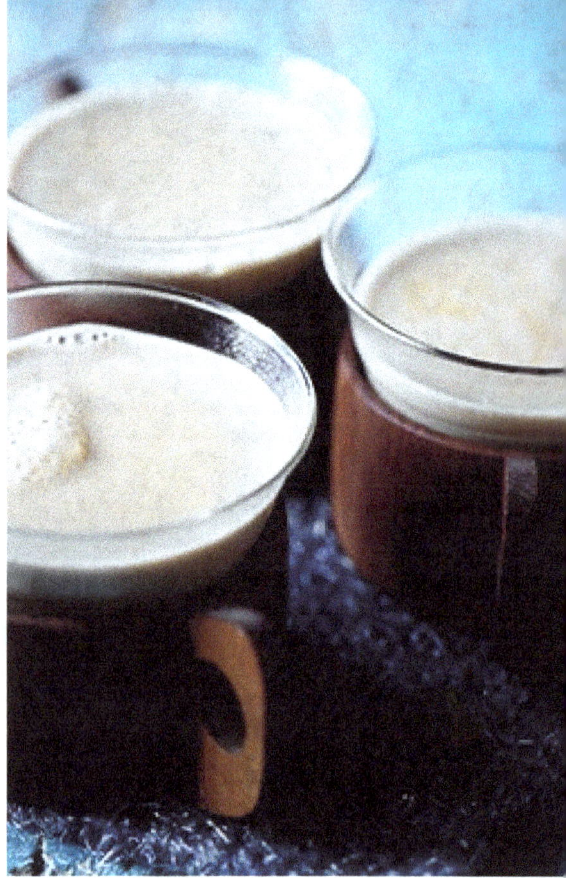

Cook Time : 10 mins

Level : Easy

Servings : Makes 2 cups

Ingredients :

- 2 mugs milk (or use almond milk)
- 2 English Breakfast tea bags
- 6 cracked cardamom pods
- ½ cinnamon stick
- a grating of fresh nutmeg
- 2 cloves
- 2-4 tsp light brown soft sugar

Method :

Heat the milk in a saucepan over a very low heat. Empty the contents of the tea bags into the pan, then add the cracked cardamom pods, cinnamon stick, nutmeg and cloves.

Chai tea

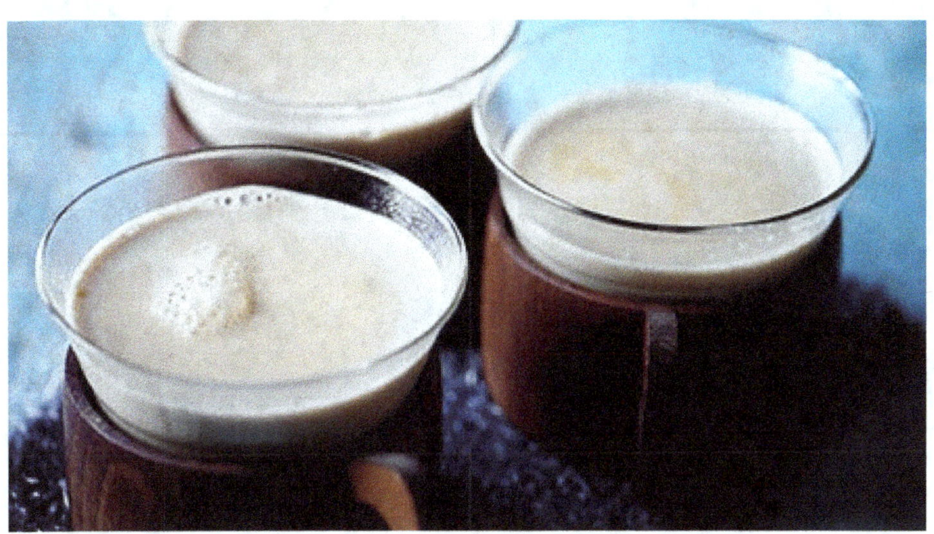

Method :

2) Sweeten with light brown soft sugar to taste (chai tea should be sweet, but use less if you like), then leave to infuse, but not boil, for 10 mins. Strain into mugs and enjoy.

Savour the comforting embrace of a spiced tea, perfectly paired with our delectable coconut chai traybake. For a vegan twist, substitute cow's milk with your preferred dairy-free alternative. We like almond milk in a chai tea, as its nutty undertones beautifully complement the warmth of the spices.

SAGE TEA

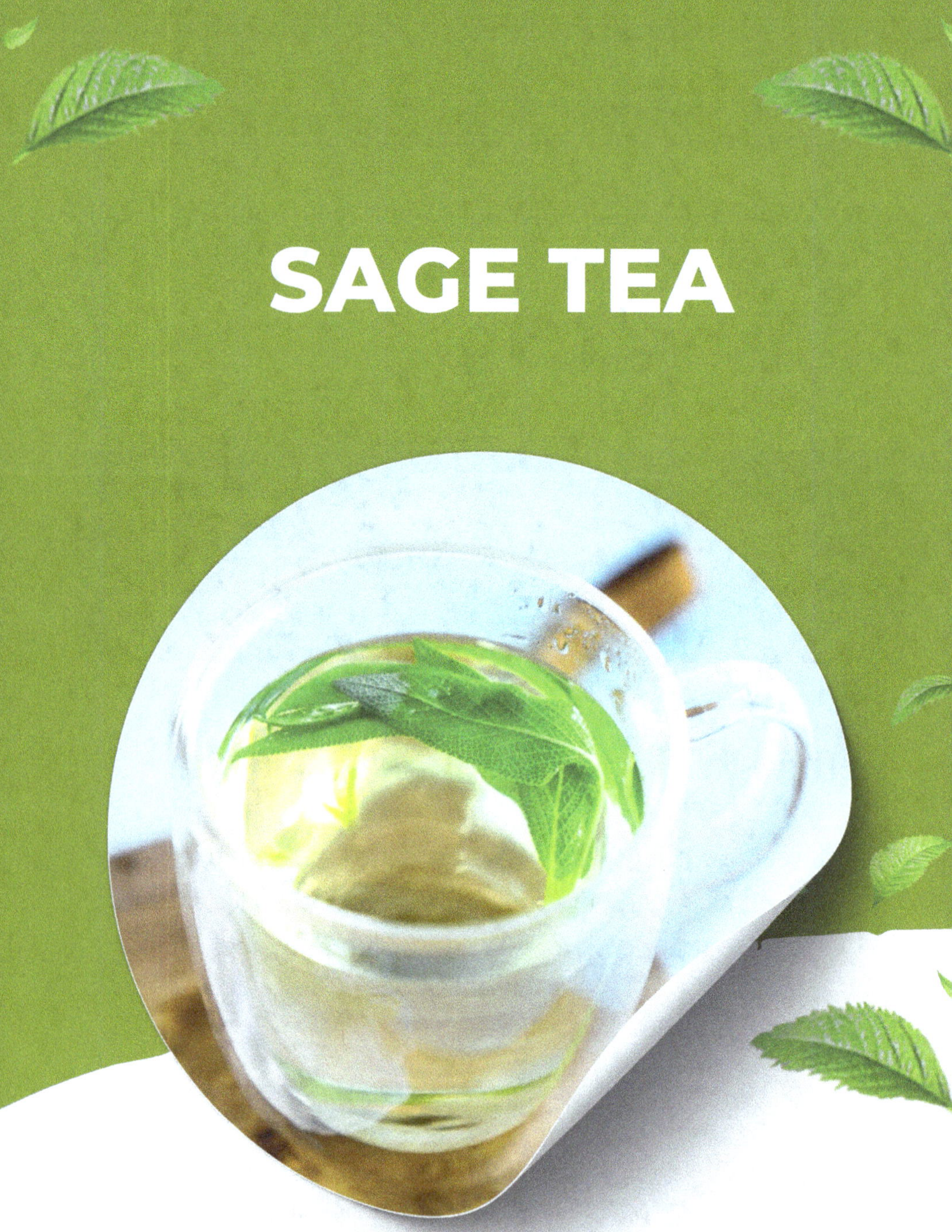

Here's how to make sage tea, a restorative herbal tea made with just boiling water and fresh sage! It's easy to make with a beautiful flavor.

Sage Tea

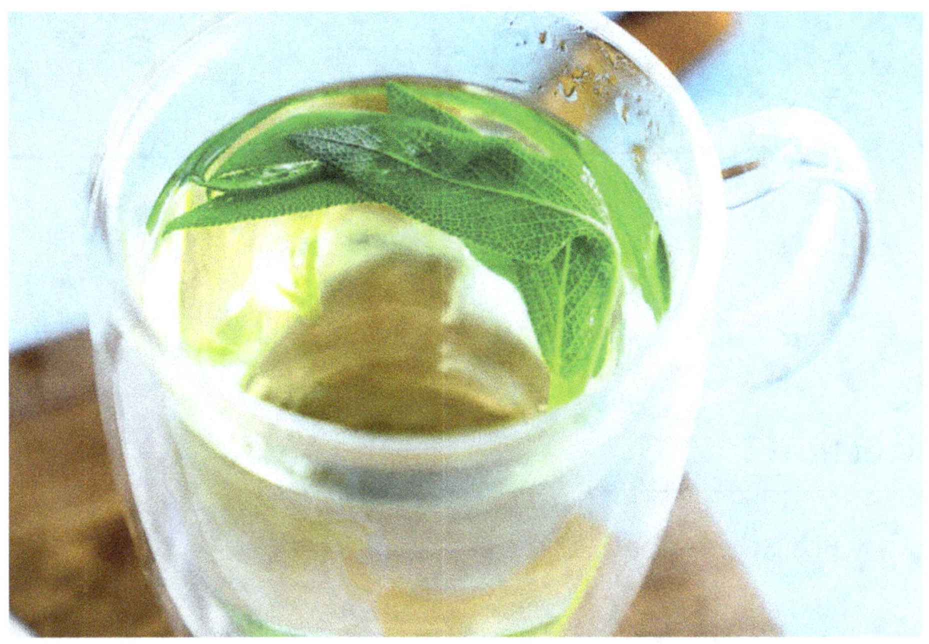

Prep Time : 5 mins

Level : Easy

Servings : 1 drink

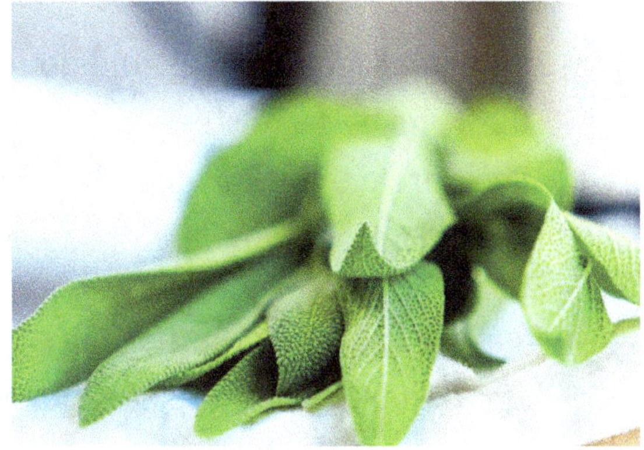

Ingredients :

- 6 fresh sage leaves, left on stem
- Boiling water
- Honey (or agave syrup for vegan)
- 1 lemon wedge

Sage Tea

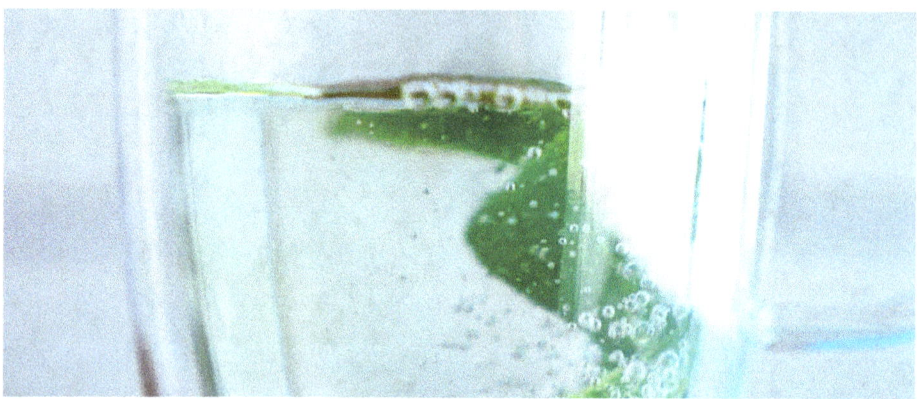

Method :

1. Bring the water to a boil.

2. Wash the sage thoroughly.

3. Place the sage in a mug, and pour over the boiling water. Allow the herbs to steep for 5 minutes. (Alternate method: If you prefer, you can also chop the sage leaves and place them in a tea strainer before steeping.)

4. Remove the sage. Stir in a drizzle of honey and a squeeze of lemon (required for the best flavor).

Let's make sage tea! It takes just 5 minutes, and this steaming cup is positively restorative. The flavor of sage herbal tea is just as you would expect: cozy and pine-forward! Add a hint of sweetener and lemon to round out the flavors, and it's positively delicious.

ICED HIBISCUS TEA

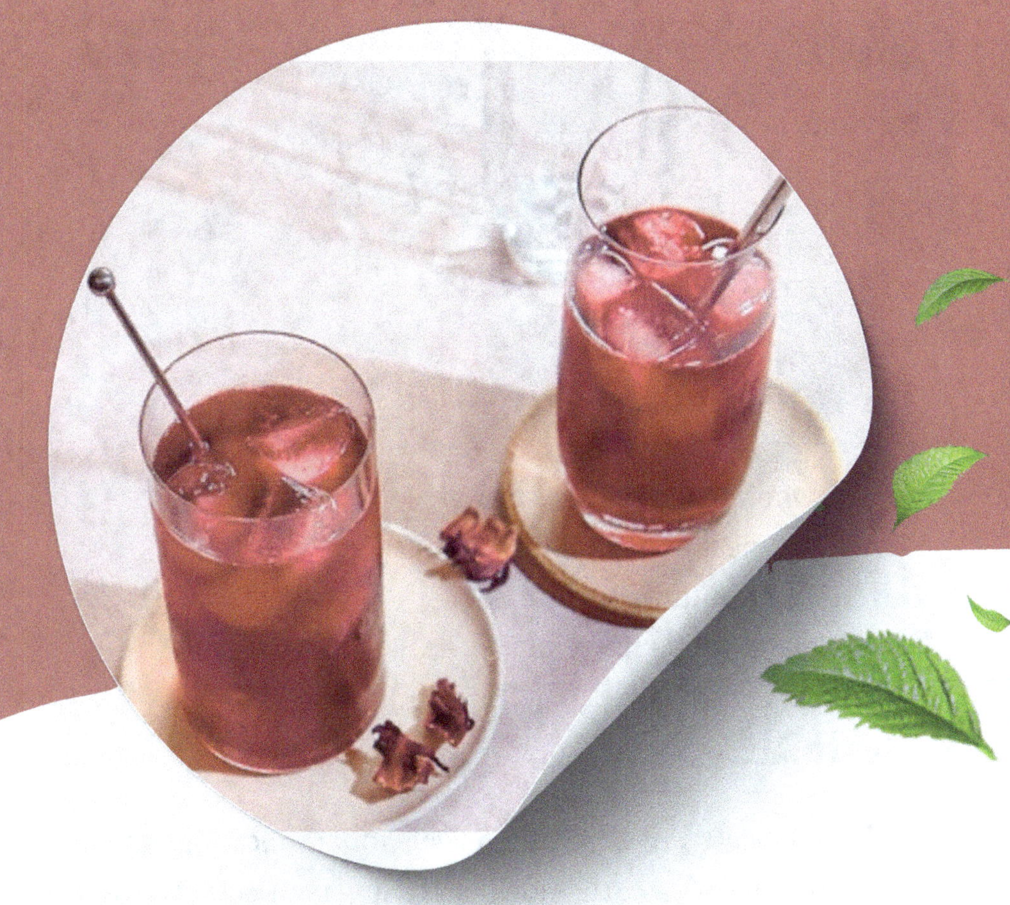

Trying to avoid sugar-laden squashes? Iced hibiscus tea is a refreshing low-sugar alternative that contains lots of beneficial compounds that act as antioxidants.

Iced hibiscus tea

Prep Time	:	5 mins
Level	:	Easy
Servings	:	Serves 2

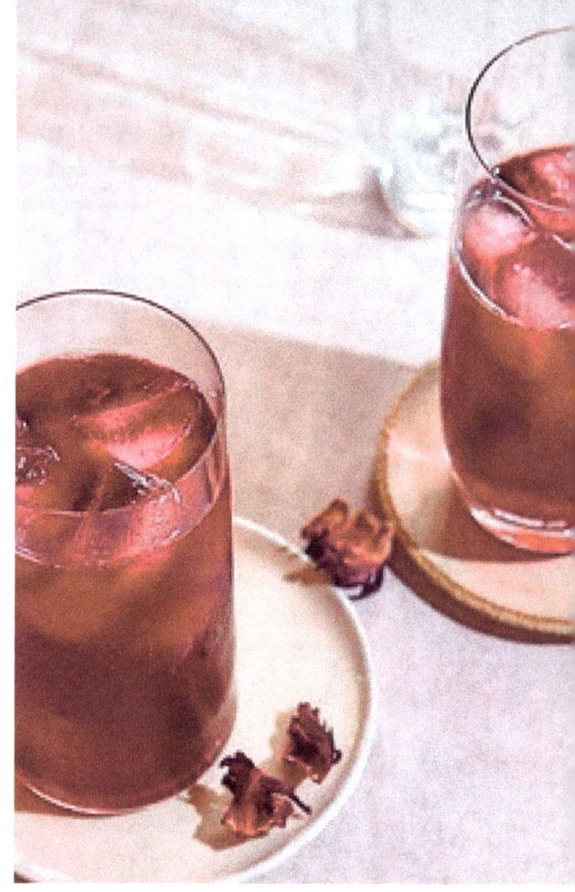

Ingredients :

- 10g whole dried hibiscus flowers
- ice and clear honey (optional), to serve

Our Most Popular Alternative

- Ultimate vanilla ice cream

Method :

1. Boil a kettle of water, then leave for around 1 min to cool to around 90C. Put the flowers in a jug, pour 500ml of the water over the flowers, then leave to steep for 16 mins. This is the optimum time and temperature for extracting the beneficial antioxidants.

Iced hibiscus tea

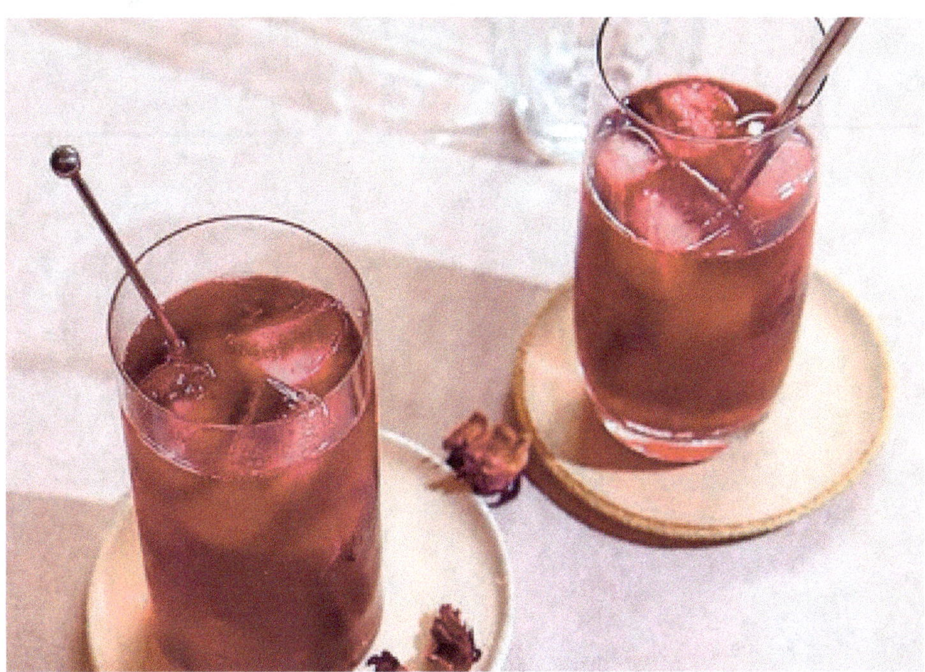

Method :

2. Strain into glasses over ice and sweeten with a litte honey, if you like.

Trying to avoid sugar-laden squashes? Iced hibiscus tea is a refreshing, low-sugar alternative that contains lots of beneficial compounds that act as antioxidants.

TURMERIC TEA

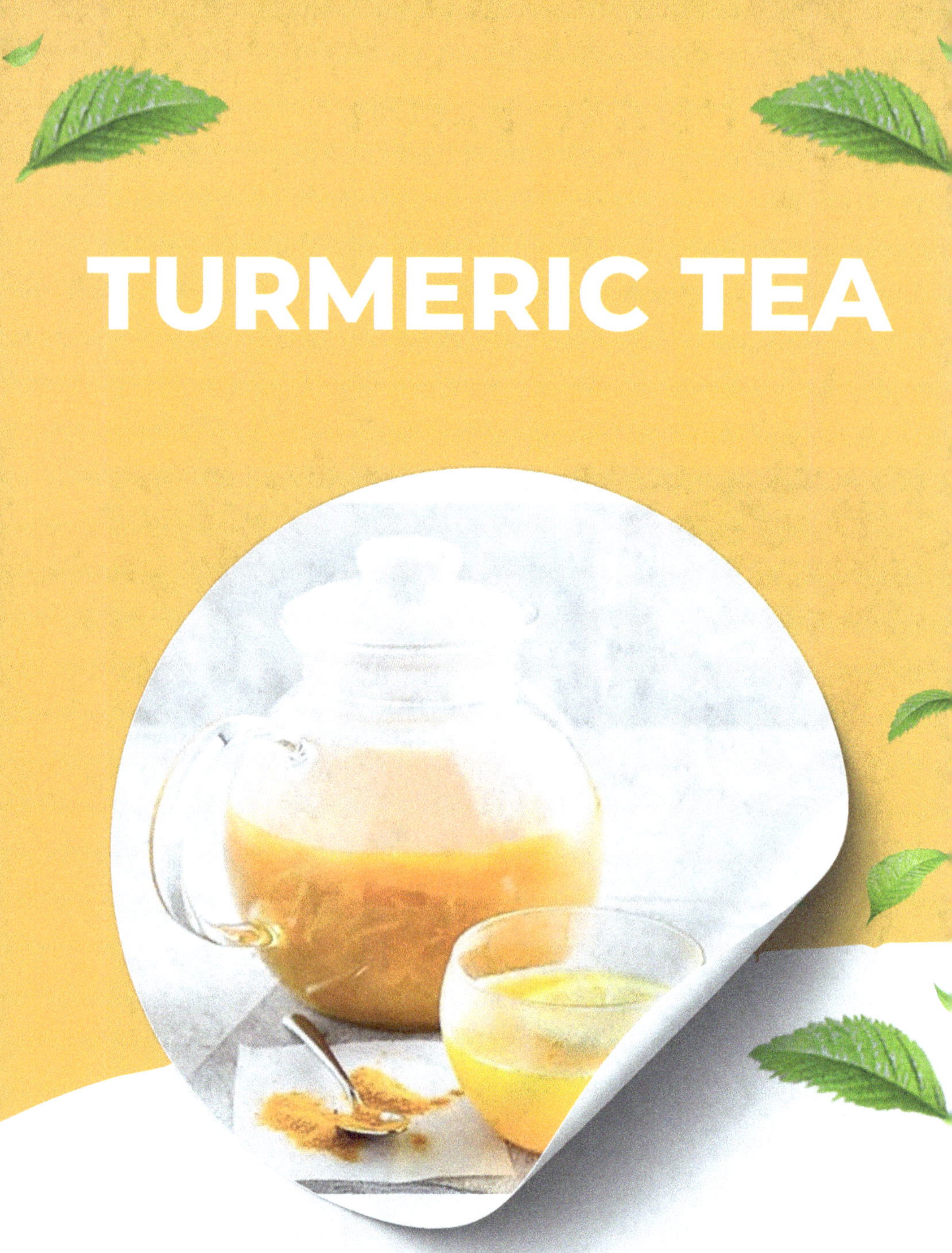

Rummage through your spice rack and dig out turmeric to make
this warming, caffeine-free tea. This bright orange spice is
popping up on menus everywhere

Turmeric tea

Cook Time : 5 mins

Level : Easy

Servings : Serves 2

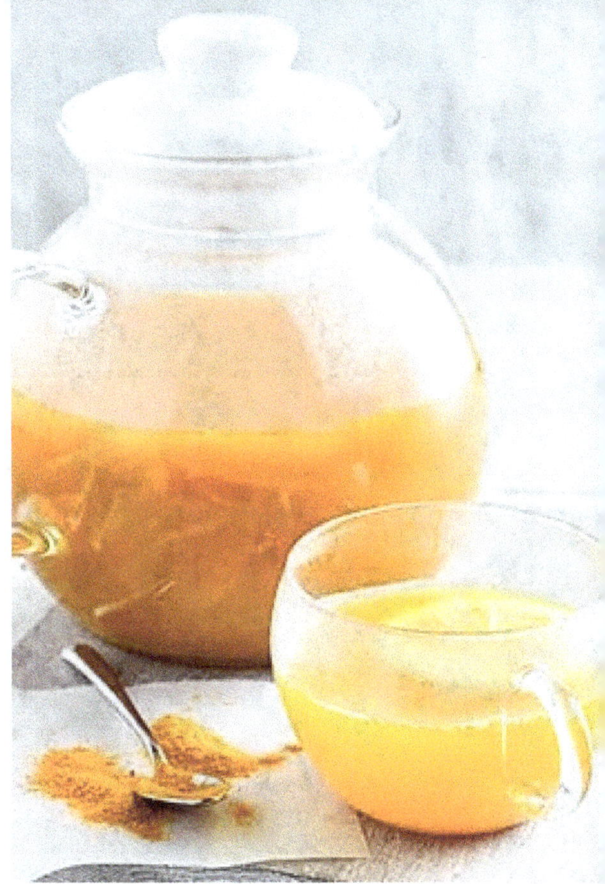

Ingredients :

- 3 heaped tsp ground turmeric
- 1 tbsp fresh grated ginger
- 1 small orange, zest pared
- honey or agave and lemon slices, to serve

Method :

1. Boil 500ml water in the kettle. Put the turmeric, ginger and orange zest in to a teapot or jug. Pour over the boiling water and allow to infuse for around 5 mins.

Chai tea

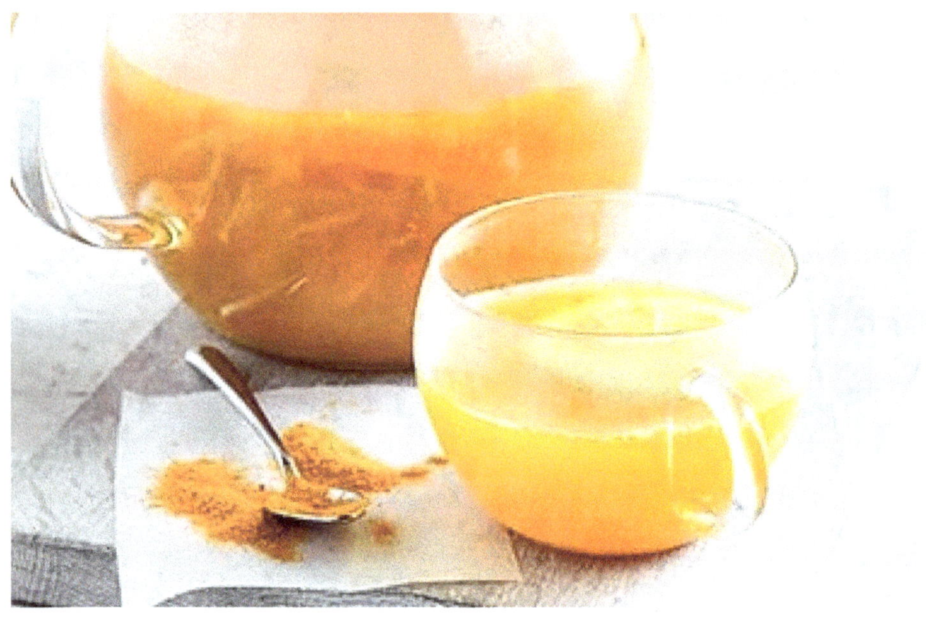

Method :

2. Strain through a sieve or tea strainer into two cups, add a slice of lemon and sweeten with honey or agave, if you like.

Explore your spice rack and try using turmeric in a soothing, caffeine-free tea. Infuse your pot with the vibrant flavours of ginger, orange, and honey for a sweet and zesty twist. Turmeric also brings numerous health benefits and aids digestion, making it an ideal choice for a post-dinner tea.

ROSEMARY & ORANGE ICED TEA

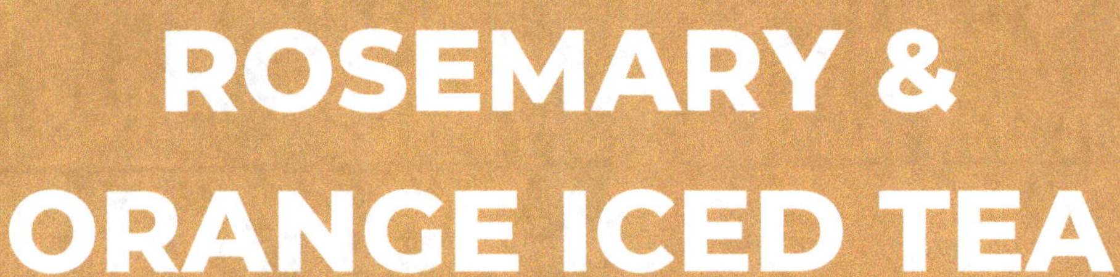

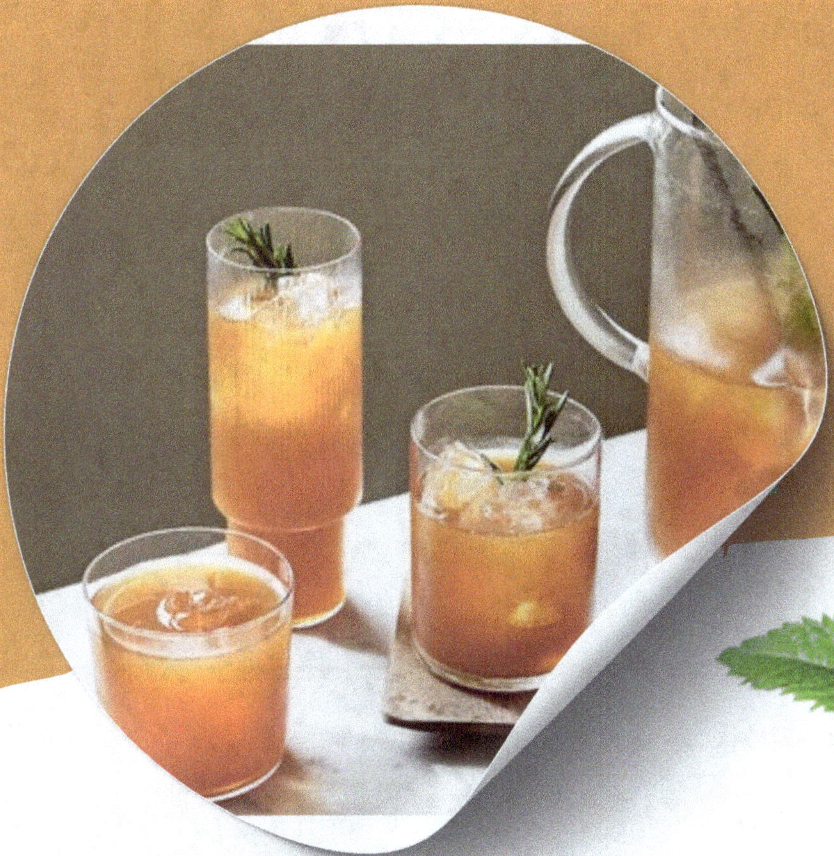

Keep cool in the summer with this aromatic infusion, with orange, tea and rosemary flavours. It's a wonderful thirst-quencher on hot, balmy days

Rosemary & orange iced tea

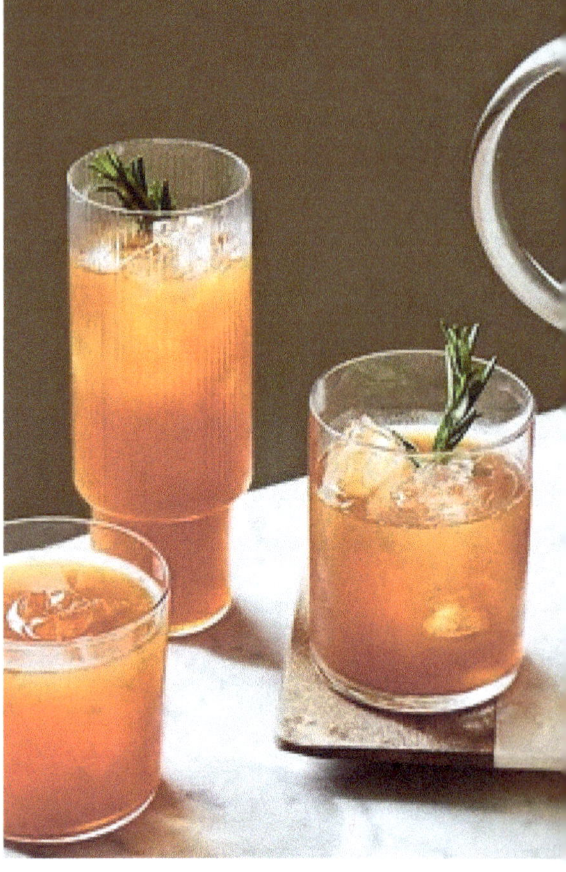

Cook Time : 5 mins

Level : Easy

Servings : Serves 4

Ingredients :

- 1 orange, juiced, zest peeled into large strips
- 3 large rosemary sprigs, plus extra to serve (optional)
- 100g golden caster sugar
- 6 teabags
- ice

Method :

1. Tip the orange peel, rosemary, sugar and 100ml water into a small saucepan and bring to a simmer. Ensuring the rosemary sprigs are submerged, cook over a low heat until the mixture has thickened slightly, about 6-8 mins. Turn off the heat. Leave to infuse for 1 hr.

Rosemary & orange iced tea

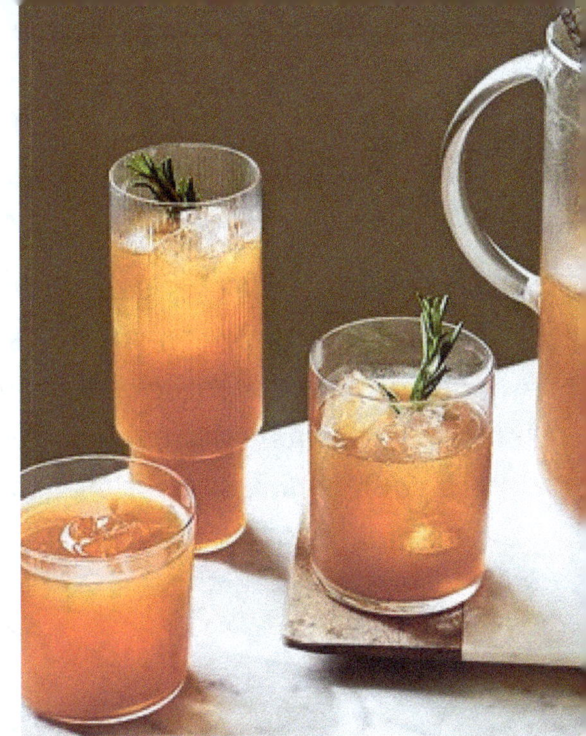

Method :

2. Put the teabags in a large heatproof jug and pour over 1 litre boiling water from the kettle. Steep for 4 mins, then discard the teabags. Leave to cool completely.

3. Stir the orange juice along with the prepared syrup into the cooled tea. Serve in highball glasses over ice. Add rosemary sprigs to garnish, if you like.

Keep cool in the summer with this aromatic infusion with orange, tea and rosemary flavours. It's a wonderful thirst-quencher on hot, balmy days.

We hope you've discovered a newfound appreciation for the simple pleasure and potential health benefits of a steaming cup of tea.

This book wouldn't be complete without you, the reader. Your passion for exploring new flavors and desire to embrace a more natural approach to wellness inspires us. We trust that the recipes within these pages will become your companions, bringing comfort, relaxation, and a touch of herbal magic to your daily life.

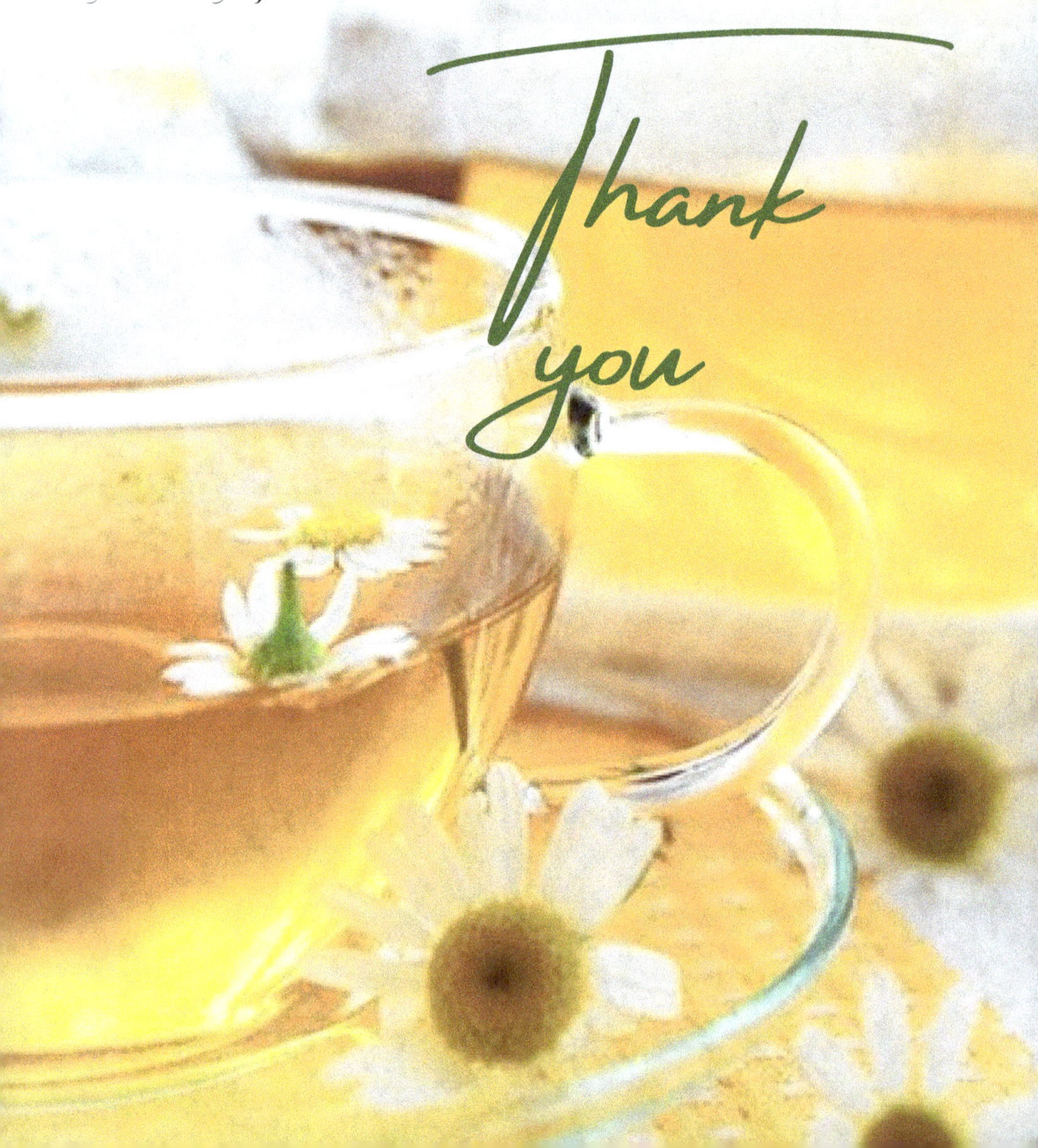

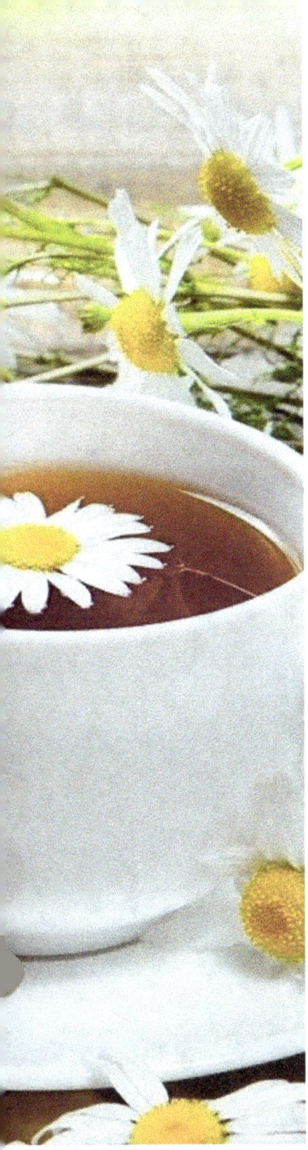

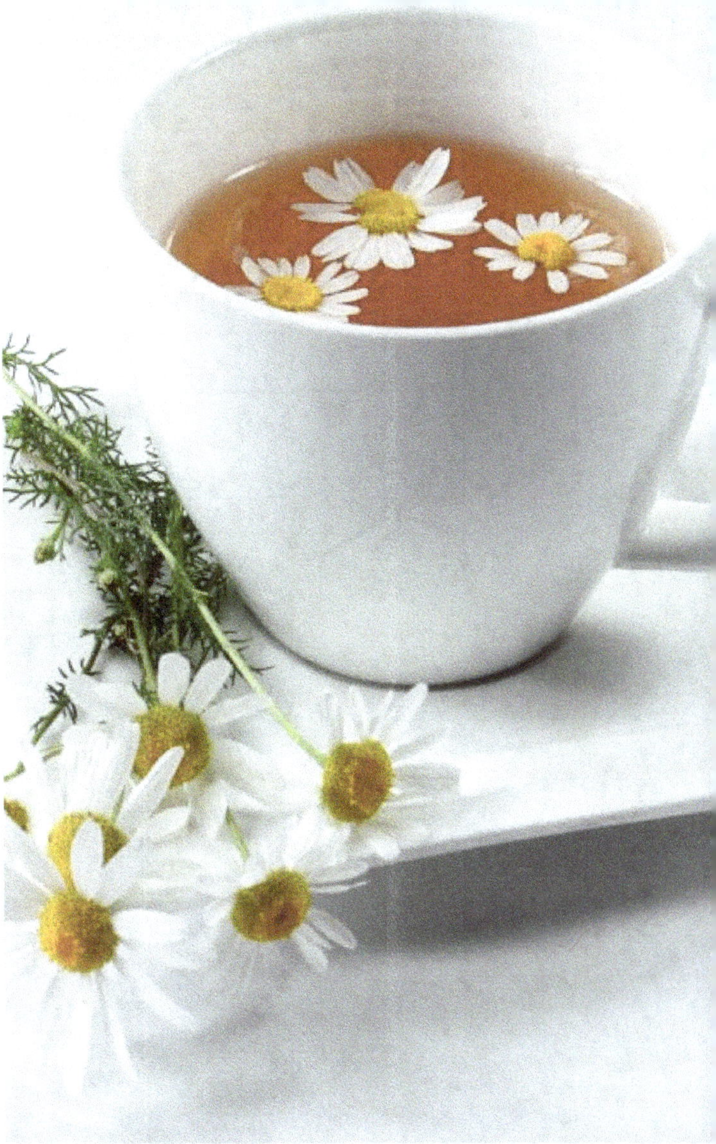

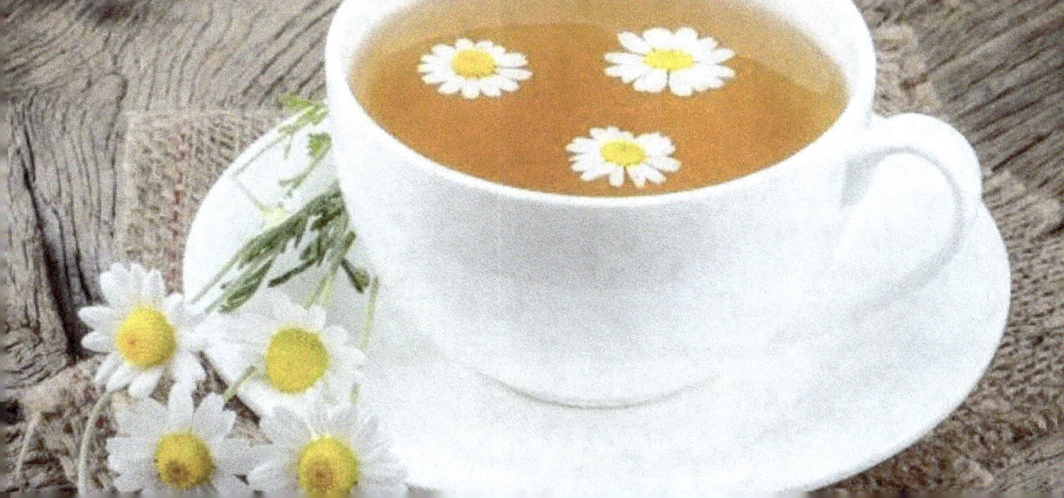

www.ingramcontent.com/pod-product-compliance
Lightning Source LLC
Chambersburg PA
CBHW071549260726
48653CB00007BA/2589